milk it:
everything you need to know about breastfeeding

**ADVICE, SOLUTIONS &
SELF-CARE FOR EVERY PARENT**

CHANTELLE CHAMPS

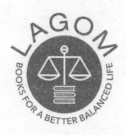

LAGOM
BOOKS FOR A BETTER BALANCED LIFE

Published by Lagom
An imprint of Bonnier Books UK
80–81 Wimpole St,
Marylebone,
London W1G 9RE

www.bonnierbooks.co.uk

Trade Paperback – 978-1-788-702-74-4
eBook – 978-1-788-702-75-1

A CIP catalogue of this book is available from the British Library.

Designed by IDSUK (DataConnection) Ltd
Printed and bound in Great Britain by Clays Ltd, Elcograf S.p.A.

1 3 5 7 9 10 8 6 4 2

The author of this book is not a health professional but a mother and the advice contained within is based on her experiences. This book is not intended to be a substitute for medical advice from a qualified clinician. If you are concerned about any aspect of breastfeeding your child, you should seek advice from your Midwife, Health Visitor or your Doctor.

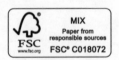

FSC
www.fsc.org

MIX
Paper from
responsible sources
FSC® C018072

To my daughters, Dakota, Tatum and Blakely. I hope this book will always be a reminder to you that you can do anything you set your mind to.

Contents

Foreword
by Kathryn Stagg, IBCLC

I came across Chantelle when she joined the Breastfeeding Twins and Triplet UK Facebook group when she was pregnant with her twins. Her first post on the group was about how she was so determined to breastfeed but that she was being told by everyone that it would be too difficult. Once several others had shared their stories, and reassured her it was totally possible, she never looked back. And despite the twins arriving a bit early and struggling a little in the early days to feed efficiently, with support from the Facebook group and local breastfeeding supporters, she did indeed fulfil her goal and breastfed the twins for over two years.

From the start Chantelle has been a voice of encouragement for so many breastfeeding mums through her Instagram account, especially twin mums. She has played a big part in normalising breastfeeding. My favourite post of hers is of her breastfeeding her twin toddlers at Disney World – this is so important to see in our society. Breastfeeding older babies is often hidden, and we have such a small percentage of babies being breastfed beyond one year in the UK, it is very rare to see. I am absolutely sure Chantelle will have encouraged so many other mums to try breastfeeding, and to continue breastfeeding for longer. And now she has put all of this enthusiasm into a book!

Milk It is a lovely, easy-to-read guide to breastfeeding and the story of Chantelle's breastfeeding journeys with her first child and then her twins. It has lots of great tips about where to find information, how to get breastfeeding going, where to get support and how to know it is working. It will be a great read for anyone expecting a baby and wanting to know a bit more about breastfeeding, how it works and whether it is something for them. Chantelle is so encouraging and enthusiastic but also empathic and honest about how it can be hard in the early days.

The take-home messages of the book are: give breastfeeding a try, it's wonderful, it can be difficult, ask for help if you need it, and any amount of breastfeeding or breast milk you can give your baby is brilliant.

Kathryn Stagg, IBCLC

About You

Your name:

....

Singleton (One)/Twins/Triplets:

....

Baby names you like:

....

Due date:

....

Birthing partner/s

....

How long you would like to breastfeed for:

....

Your ultimate breastfeeding goal:

....

How are you feeling about breastfeeding?

....

Wishes & hopes for your baby/babies:

....

Notes:

....

....

....

....

....

....

....

....

....

....

....

....

....

....

....

Hello & Welcome!

Hello, I'm Chantelle! I'm a wife to Lewis and mother to my eldest daughter Dakota (six) and my twin daughters, Tatum and Blakely (two). I'm a normal mum, the same as you. I started breastfeeding with no tools, no knowledge, and ended up experiencing one of the most amazing, rewarding journeys of my life. Due to this, I'm on a mission, mother-to-mother, to help, inspire and give confidence to other mums who want to breastfeed.

I fell in love with breastfeeding and so I learnt everything I possibly could about it. When I talk about breastfeeding, it normally ends up with me getting tearful. It's something I'm very passionate about, but I think the deep-rooted reason why I'm so emotional about the subject is because of the lack of support and knowledge I received when I wanted to breastfeed my children. I know first-hand just how important it is to have the right support and knowledge from health professionals. From speaking with hundreds of women, this is the overriding common factor of new willing mums, that they are unfortunately being let down and then struggle to breastfeed. I wanted to write a book for it to be the support you may lack and the knowledge you may not have. I want to be your friendly voice and come along with you on your breastfeeding journey, whether it be for a few days or a few years.

There is such a pressure for new mums to breastfeed, but when it comes to it, we are not given the knowledge and support we need. I was never told about any of the problems that might arise or how I could get over them. I don't know whose duty it is to speak to you about it and give you this information, but for me and many women out there, it wasn't information that was handed out to mums who wanted to breastfeed.

I breastfed my eldest daughter for 19 months and spent 27 months breastfeeding my twin daughters. Both times I really noticed a huge lack of support and knowledge given to me about breastfeeding. After having my twin daughters, I really struggled in the early days. I felt like I was on my own, with nowhere to turn, and I felt I had a fight on my hands to continue breastfeeding as I was made to feel I should be formula feeding as it was easier with multiples. Even though I had breastfed my eldest daughter successfully for 19 months and I knew what I was doing, and more importantly I knew my body knew what it was doing, I wasn't expecting breastfeeding my twins to be so challenging, with so many obstacles to cross, or how much it would take its toll on me mentally.

I think there's a common misconception that breastfeeding is going to be easy and unfortunately that just isn't always the case. So, I'm here to tell you everything I wish I'd been told and to give you all the support I wish I'd received. If you take one thing from this book, let it be that support and knowledge is power. Those two things, combined with a little determination, are the perfect recipe for a successful breastfeeding journey.

The passion I have to help women to breastfeed, or even just to inspire them to try when maybe they never wanted to before, I can feel it in my bones. I started sharing my breastfeeding journey (@chantellechamps) on Instagram in 2017 when the twins were a week old, and became inundated with messages from thousands of new mums all around the world, many of whom were feeling just like I was: alone, unsupported and looking for advice. With every mum who messaged me saying I had inspired them to breastfeed, or to continue breast-feeding, each and every one of them added fuel to my heart and I now have a burning fire inside my whole body to want to help as much as I can. I feel like I am on a mission to help as many mums as I possibly can to breastfeed successfully.

Around 81% of mums initiate breastfeeding, but then by six to eight weeks the percentage drops down to 24% for England, 17% for Wales, 13% for Northern Ireland, and the likelihood of mums still breastfeeding at six months exclusively is around 1%[1]. I believe this is because there is such a lack of support and knowledge given to new mums. Out of the mums who do decide to stop breastfeeding by six weeks, 80% of them didn't feel ready to do so, but felt like they had no other

---

[1] Infant Feeding Survey 2010 NHS National Statistics (the last UK-wide).

choice[2]. This honestly makes me feel so incredibly sad. I know from speaking with new mums that this often affects them mentally, leaving them feeling guilty that they weren't able to continue.

I want mums to know that they do have a choice and they can continue breastfeeding if they wish (not including any pre-existing medical conditions that may affect quantity of breast milk, of course). However, they are unfortunately being failed by the lack of support out there for new mums. If they were given the correct knowledge and advice, I know that our statistics in the UK would be so much higher than they are. I am certain of this because one midwife, in particular, was about to quit after six weeks of breastfeeding before she contacted me for advice and just by me giving her some information and support, she went beyond her one-year goal. If a midwife was ready to give up at six weeks because she didn't know that babies go through a major growth spurt around that time (which means babies cluster feed like crazy), how can the rest of us be expected to know this?

I was constantly being told by mums that I should write a book and as a mum myself with no prior knowledge on my first breastfeeding journey, I know what I would have liked to have read. I don't want to overwhelm you with the science; this book is for mums who have made the decision they would like to breastfeed and I'm going to

---

[2] https://www.ncbi.nlm.nih.gov/pmc/articles/PMC4494694/

hopefully be able to help them achieve this. I want mums to feel supported when they may not otherwise have been, I want them to feel confident in their knowledge, and most importantly, I want them to feel inspired and confident that they can feed their babies in the way they want to, when they want to and where they want to. My book will be with you every step of the way when you doubt yourself, when you're having a bad day and when you have problems you want to overcome. I want you to feel like you are connecting with me, another mum who has been there and overcome it. If I can do it, you can do it, and we are in this together.

You can use this book to figure out what's best for you. Read about my journey with breastfeeding and gain all of the knowledge I found, and then remain safe in the knowledge that whatever you choose, you are doing just fine! You do what is right for you and your baby!

Dear Mums . . .

Hey, Mama!

I'm guessing if you've picked up this book, you are either pregnant and would like to breastfeed, or you have recently had your baby and are in the early stages of breastfeeding. Well, let me tell you, you've come to the right place. I have been where you are right now and I successfully breastfed my eldest daughter for 19 months and have just finished breastfeeding my twin daughters for 27 months. Unfortunately, I didn't receive much help, support or knowledge from health professionals, which meant I had to take matters into my own hands. Everything in this book is a product of my own research and hard work, with extra know-how from the amazing lactation consultant, Kathryn Stagg, IBCLC.

Looking back on both of my breastfeeding journeys, the best way I can describe them is that it's like climbing a mountain. If you decided one day you wanted to climb Mount Everest, the first thing you would do is research. You could not go into something like that completely unprepared, you would fuel your brain with knowledge on how to get to the top of that mountain, so you knew exactly what to expect, and when to expect it. You would also find out if there was anything you could buy to make your journey easier, as preparing yourself before you start, well, that's winning half the battle. Once you start your journey up the mountain, you are likely to come across some pitfalls. But you have already prepared yourself, so you already know they might come up, and more importantly, you know how to overcome them to successfully carry on your journey. Then, and this is the best bit, once you reach the top of the mountain, you are over the hard part, you've successfully made it, all of the 'training' before your journey started has paid off and you overcame all the tough stages you knew were likely to happen. This is when you get to take in the breath-taking view. And the best part of your journey has only just begun. You get to look back and think, Yes, I'm a badass, I've smashed this and done what I set out to do!

I'm here to help you prepare for your breastfeeding journey, so you can reach the best part and maybe even fall in love with breastfeeding, just like I did. I wasn't an expert, I started out with no knowledge and no experience. I didn't take to breastfeeding initially, I had no clue what I was doing, but, funnily enough, my babies had never done it before so we had to learn together. With my first child, there were many things I had to overcome and I had lots of last-minute researching to do, only adding to my stress. The second time around, I knew I had to do my research, especially as I was having twins, if I wanted to have another successful journey. Of course, I still came up against problems but when faced with health professionals trying to push me to formula feed the twins, I was fuelled with knowledge and confidence that I knew I could breastfeed – I knew (within reason) I could get over most problems and I knew my body was made to do this. Did I have times at the start of our journey when I wanted to quit? Absolutely I did, but on the tough days I never lost sight that tomorrow could be my best day, and here I am now, telling my story and hoping to inspire and give confidence to as many women as I can.

I am hoping I can help as many mums as possible to be able to reach the best part, the top of the mountain. It will be an amazing journey, a lot of hard work in the beginning, but the rewards are endless. So, let me finish off by saying a massive congratulations on your pregnancy/newborn/s and a big good luck on your journey. You are not alone and we can do this together!

Chantelle xx

My Story

Throughout these pages, I have written about my personal experiences where relevant. I want this book to not feel like a textbook with no feeling behind it – I want to give you advice as I would my friends. So, I've been an open book as much as I can (pardon the pun!). I want to start by telling you the story of my pregnancy, my labour, my breastfeeding experience from start to finish – all my struggles and my triumphs. I felt like I didn't just want to write this book, I needed to – a need I felt with my whole body, from head to toe. Hopefully, after you read my story, you will understand why.

In January 2017, I had an almost three-year-old daughter (Dakota) and me and my husband Lewis had been trying for baby number two for a few months. Lots of ovulation tests, reading books, changing my diet, meditating (I am one of those women that cannot go with the flow and relax!) and a few months later, I had the faintest line appear on a pregnancy test a few days before my missed period. I was pregnant and we were expecting our second child! We were absolutely over the moon, but at the same time I had just found out my grandad Colin (Cole Cole), my best friend, was dying. He had mesothelioma, which is an asbestos-related cancer. So, the news of me being pregnant was bittersweet.

Then, the day my period was due, it started: hyperemesis gravidarum, HG for short. Some of you may have heard about this and others may not. Normally, when I tell people they say, 'Oh, what Princess Kate had?' HG is not morning sickness; it is extreme, relentless sickness, anytime of the day and anything can start it off. It is completely debilitating and leaves you mentally and physically unwell. I had it when I was pregnant with my eldest, Dakota, and was hospitalised a lot and this second time around, I had her to take care of as well.

The sound of my daughter doing a wee in her potty would set my sickness off, her cuddling me would set it off, and once I started, I just didn't stop – until normally I ended up in hospital with a cocktail of drugs running through my veins. Sometimes I couldn't even swallow my own saliva without throwing it back up.

I had a scan at nine weeks, when they told me I was expecting one baby, and one baby only. Because I had been so ill, twice as bad as my first pregnancy (which didn't even seem possible), I said, 'Please check and make sure I'm not having twins.' I left the hospital feeling happy it was the one baby, the thought of two just scared me so much!

In between weeks 9 and 13 of pregnancy, my sickness got worse and I spent most of my time in my bedroom with the lights off, television off, blinds closed. I couldn't take calls from my friends, I couldn't sit up. The smell of food cooking would set me off, there were days when I would just have to lay flat on the bed with my eyes closed, trying to block out how nauseous I felt. It was relentless, depressing, isolating and just so, so tough on me, physically and mentally, which had a huge impact on my daughter. Lewis still had to work, so he had to call upon family members to take care of me and Dakota because it was physically impossible for me to be able to look after our daughter.

One day my sickness started again. I was 11 weeks pregnant and knew this time in particular was going to end up in a hospital admission. Normally with an IV drip and anti-sickness drugs through the IV, it would ease, because I wouldn't be able to throw the medication back up. This time it was different – I still didn't stop throwing up! They tried all different kinds of drug, my dehydration level wasn't getting any better (even after eight IV drips). On day 3 in hospital, I became absolutely desperate – I remember crying and begging the nurses to do something, there must be something we hadn't tried that could stop this hell. A doctor came round to check on me and I told her, 'I have 24 hours left in me and if I'm still throwing up this time tomorrow, I'm going to have to speak to my husband about a termination. I cannot physically or mentally carry on.' I was heart-broken just saying those words and writing them now brings tears to my eyes.

The next day, during what felt like a miracle, my sickness finally settled down. I went to the toilet and noticed I was bleeding, and then the panic took over my body. The guilt I felt for what I had said the day before will stay with me forever. I thought I was losing my baby. I spoke with the nurse, who thought I had pulled something inside from the amount of times I'd been sick and that was the reason for my bleeding.

A few days later, I had a second scan and that was when I found out the reason I was bleeding. When I looked at the screen, I saw two heads: I was expecting twins. I kept giggling and crying on and off for the whole hour Lewis and I were in the scan room and my overriding emotion was of completely crapping myself, mixed in with some excitement and straight back to, 'WHAT THE HELLLLL?' The moment I found out, after a few choice swear words, one of the first things I said was, 'I won't be able to breastfeed.' Having fallen in love with breastfeeding after doing so with my eldest daughter, my excitement at being able to breastfeed again and having that connection with another little human was so high. In that moment I felt like that was being taken away from me and I would never get to experience breastfeeding again.

We left the hospital and immediately drove round to our families to tell them all the exciting news, that we weren't expecting one baby, but in fact two babies. This is when the comments started straight away: 'Oh, you're not thinking of breastfeeding twins, are you? Your boobs will be down by your ankles!' with a lot of laughing, all at my expense. Everyone knew how I felt about breastfeeding, the love I had for it, and I had already experienced the fight some of them gave me because I breastfed past six months with my first child. Now I had just found out I was having twins (which was scary enough) and already the judgements came flooding in. I went home even more determined that I wanted to find out if breastfeeding twins was even possible. How dare anyone comment and take the mickey out of my love for breastfeeding my child instead of encouraging me and supporting me on the prospect of breastfeeding my twins; they showed me nothing but ridicule and criticism. Little did they know, they were just fuelling my fire!

I started researching online and found out women can breastfeed multiples (some of you may be reading this and think, *Of course you can breastfeed more than one baby*, but I genuinely had no clue, I certainly didn't know anyone breastfeeding twins). Thankfully, I found the Facebook group 'Breastfeeding Twins and Triplets UK', which had thousands and thousands of mums to multiples successfully breastfeeding their children exclusively. I could never have felt more empowered and inspired by these women. *If they can breastfeed more than one baby, then so can I*, I thought to myself. That was my decision made and from then on out, no one was going to change that.

When I told the same family members, who had ridiculed me, that I had done my research and it was my decision, they started an argument with me, telling me it just wasn't possible. It was coming from a good place, but they were debating with me even though I had made an informed and educated decision, and it was my body and my babies. After that, I had lots of rows about it, but there was no way I was going to have my decision changed by anyone. I was of course nervous and scared; I knew it was going to be incredibly hard, not only physically but mentally. I was already nervous, with hormones flying around, and going through a huge mental strain because my grandad was dying. It affected me deeply. At this time my grandad Cole Cole was in the hospital having bad side effects from his chemotherapy, so me and Dakota would visit him daily. We would talk about me breastfeeding the twins and he would encourage me and say how proud he was of me.

Thirty-five weeks into my pregnancy, my waters broke. You don't wait until you're having contractions with twins to go to hospital, you go straight there to be monitored. In both of my labours, my body just didn't dilate very well – I get to a certain point and no matter how long or how many contractions later, I don't dilate any more. I have to have a hormone drip to speed up contractions to get me to do so.

I was taken to theatre, and although I wanted a natural birth, they said it was for the best to already be in theatre just in case they had trouble with twin two, who was now breech. As a precaution, I was set up for an emergency C-section (caesarean). I had an epidural and was on a C-section bed, which let me tell you, is not the best position to be in giving birth naturally as I was at completely the wrong angle for pushing and it just felt wrong. I wasn't pushing for long before they used forceps for me to give birth to Twin 1, my daughter Tatum.

After that, it's a bit of a blur. I remember someone saying they had hold of Twin 2 inside my womb, but my cervix was closing, so instead of remaining at 10cm dilated, I was now at 8cm. Someone explained that if I gave birth naturally, the outcome for Twin 2 could be fatal and it was crucial to get her out as quickly and safely as possible with an emergency C-section. I had been allowed three birthing partners – my husband, my mum (Zelda) and my sister Nikita – and they were all told to leave except for Lewis. And then in came a lot of other health professionals.

They topped up my epidural but I could still feel them touching my stomach and they said I would have to have a general anaesthetic if I could feel them touching me. At this point, they told Lewis he had to leave too. He gave me a kiss and left, but I couldn't bring myself to say goodbye to him – I honestly thought if I said goodbye, I would never wake up. After thinking about this, I immediately said, 'No, cut me open, I'm not in any pain. I can feel you touching me but I'm not in any pain, I do not want to be put to sleep and I want you to go ahead straight away.' In this moment I remember going back to my hypnobirthing training – I took myself to another place, calmed my breathing and relaxed. I do not remember when my husband came back in or giving birth to Twin 2 – another daughter, Blakely. The next memory I have is of Lewis suddenly being there and I had given birth to both of our daughters, who were across the room to me. My midwife asked if I would like to meet and have a cuddle with Blakely and immediately my first instinct was that I needed to breastfeed!

Everything had gone wrong and I felt an overwhelming instinct that I needed to get it back together. I had never felt so un-motherly, I needed to feel like a new mum who had just given birth. We had a little feed, although my nipple just seemed so large for Blakely's tiny mouth. I was wheeled to recovery and finally reunited with my mum and Nikita. I remember saying to them, 'I do not feel like a mum at all.'

At this point I was completely out of it on morphine! I was breastfeeding Blakely on my left and being milked by complete strangers on my right (not random people, don't worry, but a new set of midwives I had just met!). Because the girls were premature, they had already tested them and said their blood sugars were low. I can remember one of them saying, 'You have ten minutes and if you haven't expressed enough milk, we're going to give them formula.' I was also told I had to produce 15ml (3 teaspoons) of colostrum every three hours – this doesn't sound a lot, but for someone who has just given birth, this is a lot of milk to be expected. Low blood sugar is when your baby's demand for glucose is greater than its supply, something that is common in preterm births (babies born at less than 37 weeks). Your baby gets glucose from the lactose that's in your milk and colostrum. (Colostrum is the first milk women produce when they give birth, before milk production begins. It is filled with nutrients to help growth and fight diseases in infants.) Breast milk has a higher carbohydrate content and large amounts of lactose, more than formula, but my body just wasn't producing enough milk. A few factors come into play here: the fact my daughters were premature, that I had a traumatic birth and also a C-section.

I remember feeling so upset, thinking, *I've just given birth, which went wrong. I do not feel like a mum, I'm desperate to breastfeed my babies* – I could just see my breastfeeding journey disappearing right in front of my eyes. The biggest problem for me was there was no breastfeeding specialist on duty, I only had a midwife I had just met after giving birth telling me these demands without much of an explanation or plan in place. In situations like this, when there is low blood sugar, formula top-ups can help when you cannot produce enough milk or if you haven't previously expressed some before your birth. I always felt someone should have explained to me exactly the ins and outs of it all – obviously to them it is probably something they see often, but to a new mum after a traumatic birth who didn't know anything about blood sugar and hadn't been forewarned that this was common in early births, it was so stressful and upsetting. I felt like I was failing my babies once again, even though it was just another challenge to overcome and I would still have been able to breastfeed. For me it was highly stressful and emotional and not how I imagined my breastfeeding journey would start.

I always felt like my desire to breastfeed my babies was an inconvenience to the hospital staff. Some made comments about it not being possible to breastfeed twins exclusively, which I knew was not true, and others told me to combi-feed for ease. But my wish was to breastfeed exclusively. I knew I was capable as I had given birth before and I also knew I was going to do it, no matter what anyone said. I told the paediatrician and nurses that I desperately wanted to breastfeed and there were no two ways about it, but I felt like I wasn't being given a choice or options. So eventually I gave in, but I made them put a plan in place and breastfeeding directly from me always had to come first. I did request donor breast milk as you need smaller amounts of breast milk to help blood sugar levels than formula, but my hospital did not store donor milk, so it had to be formula top-ups until I started producing more milk.

The plan was for me to hand express every few hours, put my babies on my breasts first, and then to top up with my expressed breast milk with the difference made up with formula. They wanted to give my daughters the milk in bottles, which I refused – I didn't want them getting used to a bottle and then not being able to latch onto my breasts properly, potentially hindering our breastfeeding journey further, so it was either syringe or tube feeding. I cannot remember how we got to the decision but the girls ended up having tubes through their noses and down their throats so they would get the colostrum I had hand expressed and also the formula top-ups. I had a midwife come in and explain to me the more formula the girls had the more their stomachs would stretch and I would then be playing catch-up with my milk supply to keep up with their stomachs expanding. You will read further in the book how breastfeeding works on a demand and supply basis (*see also* pages 53–65).

Although I was so thankful for someone actually explaining something to me, I felt even more like I was under pressure to perform: my boobs needed to do their job. I had my alarm set every three hours around the clock: I was a woman on a mission!

A few days after the births, at around 1am, a nurse came in to feed the girls. I had expressed the most milk I had expressed earlier, 30ml, and it was sat waiting on the table next to me. The nurse came in and went straight to express the formula into the girls' feeding tubes. This was not the plan, this was not what I had agreed to, they were meant to feed directly from me, then my expressed colostrum, then the formula top-up. I felt like I had a light-bulb moment – this woman did not seem to care about my breastfeeding desire, or what I wanted; I felt she just wanted to tick some boxes and move on to the next patient. I am sure in her head she didn't consciously think this way, but it was sure how I felt at the time. Looking back now I think she may have not been informed of our plan, but either way I was left feeling like my desire to breastfeed my daughters was not being met. I remember as clear as day, I said to her, 'No, this is not the plan, this is not what I want.' I broke down crying and then asked her to leave. Then I looked at my little pot of bright yellow colostrum sitting there – I had been so proud of the volume of milk I had produced and it was just going to be discarded. From that moment the girls didn't have any more formula: they had been given numerous blood tests around the clock and their last blood sugar test after solely breastfeeding was finally above the average line – they were now producing enough glucose in their blood.

I know reading this, you may not understand why this affected me so much, but even writing it, I have tears in my eyes! After having to convince health professionals I could breastfeed my babies, I was exhausted mentally and physically after the birth. But I am a much stronger person because of it. I had gone my whole life not wanting to offend anyone, always doing as I was told (not even joking, I didn't get one detention in school). Motherhood has taught me that I can stand up for myself and what I want for me and my children and – to follow my gut instinct. The reason I felt so assured of my decision to breastfeed was because I had researched and knew exactly what had to be done to ensure a successful breastfeeding journey.

After leaving the hospital, breastfeeding the twins was not exactly plain sailing. I had lots of ups and downs in the early days. We had issues with our second twin, Blakely, as she had reached 10 per cent weight loss (10 per cent is the maximum amount of weight hospital teams like babies to lose, more explained later[1]). On day 6 after leaving hospital, I was back in again: Blakely had reached 10.1 per cent loss, now weighing just under 1.5kg [3lb 5oz]. Once again, I had the overwhelming feeling of failure, I felt sick and cried the whole way to the hospital.

---

[1] www.nct.org.uk/baby-toddler/feeding/common-concerns/my-baby-not-gaining-weight

When we got there, Blakely's temperature was so low, they thought the thermometer had broken! Straight away, they admitted her and I completely broke down – I felt like I couldn't even do the simple thing of keeping my baby warm. I requested they also check Tatum and as she was also under the normal temperature, she was admitted too. Both had to go in an incubator and were only allowed out for feeding. I completely blamed myself, but the reality was that they were premature and had no fat to regulate their temperature (just the short car journey to hospital might have been enough to cause the significant drop in their temperatures).

I was told I had to write down every time they fed and for how long. Again, I felt like I was under scrutiny and had this huge pressure on me. Thankfully, Blakely didn't lose any more weight and after a few days, we were allowed home again, but it felt a little like déjà vu. I was so anxious for every midwife check-up and couldn't wait to be discharged.

The first six weeks were by far the toughest, especially because my grandad passed away the day the twins turned one month old. I was mentally not OK, struggling with grief, new mum life to twin babies and breastfeeding around the clock. I remember the six-week growth spurt and how my target was to get past this stage. If I could get over that, the mammoth cluster feeding and everything else I had experienced in my breastfeeding journey up until this point, I knew I could truly conquer anything breastfeeding was going to throw at me, and I did it. I stuck to my guns, didn't let anyone influence my decisions, and put a lot of hard work into it. It's probably one of the proudest moments of anything I have ever done to date. Our breastfeeding journey continued until the twins were 27 months old, and I cannot even begin to tell you how much I miss it.

FUN FACT

Your baby can smell you out because of your breast milk

Your baby will start to recognise your scent before they are even born, and afterwards, will be able to pick you out up to two feet away just from your scent. Your smell is a part of the amniotic fluid which nourishes your child in the womb, so they will know your breast milk scent and taste almost immediately. If your baby is in any pain, they can be relieved by just the smell of your milk as it is unique to you.[2]

[2] www.breastfeedingrose.org/incredible-facts-about-breastfeeding-for-mommy-baby/

I'M NOT TELLING YOU
IT'S GOING TO BE EASY,
I'M TELLING YOU IT'S
GOING TO BE WORTH IT.

Feed Your Babies How You Want

My first and best piece of advice I could give any new mum is to feed your babies how you want, not how other people want you to. If you're reading this and you're pregnant, then you may have started speaking to friends and family about how you would like to feed your baby and hopefully however you decide, they will fully support you.

Unfortunately, this isn't always the case. I feel like this is something really important to talk about, as I know a lot of pregnant women and new mums are having this same argument with the closest people in their life. In both of my pregnancies, I was constantly met with judgements and unwanted opinions from people who loved me. They all wanted the best for me, but they added so much stress and anxiety to my pregnancies, filling my head with self-doubt, which is not what I wanted when I had made the decision of how I wanted to feed my baby. I stuck to my guns and exclusively breastfed all three of my children, and the people who didn't think I should breastfeed ended up respecting me so much for feeding my babies in the way I wanted to and not how they thought I should.

Don't let anyone tell you how to feed your children. You might get to the end of this book and decide you do not want to breastfeed and that is completely fine, of course. Or you might decide that you want to give breastfeeding a try, or that you want to breastfeed exclusively for two years. However YOU decide to feed your children is the right decision for you and that's the main thing to learn.

People who may try to persuade you not to breast-feed are usually coming from a good place and mean well. They are giving you the advice that they think is best, but unfortunately, it is likely an uneducated opinion. But because the unwanted opinion is coming from someone who cares for you, it's all too easy to take it in and misinterpret the information you are being given. It's so important to work out whether you are being given an uneducated opinion or educated advice, as they can get confused for one another. Unless you know someone has knowledge about breastfeeding, it's always so important to do your own research so you can tackle any negative, uneducated opinions and then make a fully informed decision.

The best ways to tackle negativity I found are as follows:

Educate

As I said above, most people who make negative comments on breastfeeding are probably not educated on the subject. Maybe try and see this as an opportunity to teach someone – it might not necessarily change their view, but you will feel better for providing them with facts, as opposed to their opinions.

Question

When people come out with their uninformed comments, ask them, 'Why are you so against breastfeeding?' or even, 'Why do you have a problem with me feeding my baby how I want to?' Most of the time they will probably not be able to answer. If they took a few minutes to actually think about the questions, I bet they wouldn't even know why. Also ask for evidence for their comments. Do they have the science to back up their opinions?

One of the classic answers I received when I asked these questions was, 'It's going to be too much for you', so I would reply that it was down to me to decide and I would see when the time came. Whether a baby is breast- or bottle fed, they need to be fed! Personally, I always found breastfeeding easier compared to the thought of bottle feeding. When my girls woke up in the night, I didn't have to get out of bed, I just popped them on and then off without having to leave the bedroom.

Honesty

Be brutally honest and let people know how you feel about their comments. A lot of women keep their feelings bottled up, including myself. As I am writing this, I can feel my blood boiling as this was a constant battle through both of my pregnancies and it still boggles my mind today how anyone could think they have a right to try and dictate how you feed YOUR child. I did end up saying,

'I don't mean to be rude, but this is MY baby! You can comment as much as you like, but you're wasting your breath as I am going to feed MY baby how I want to. I have done enough research and am happy with the decision I have made for me and my family.' I'm not saying this is going to work miracles, but it's worth a go.

FUN FACT

Breastfeeding helps you lose weight

If you breastfeed, you will burn around 500 extra calories a day. Breastfeeding also releases the hormones that trigger your uterus to return to its pre-baby size faster. When your baby starts feeding, you can actually feel uterine contractions as the uterus starts to shrink. When I was breastfeeding the twins, I burnt around 1,000 calories a day![1]

---

[1] 'Off to the Best Start', Start4Life, Unicef leaflet: https://www. unicef.org.uk/babyfriendly/baby-friendly-resources/breastfeeding-resources/off-to-the-best-start/

I AM ALL MY LITTLE ONE NEEDS.

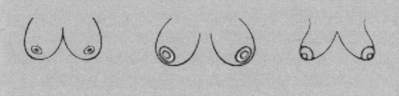

PART 1

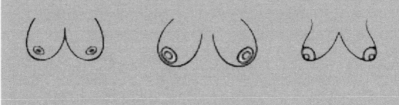

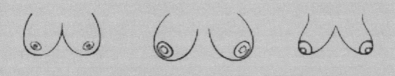

PREGNANCY & BIRTH

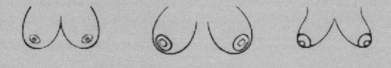

1

Preparing for Your Breastfeeding Journey

I wanted to start this book from the very beginning: the moment you find out you're pregnant and are thinking about giving breastfeeding a go. You may be reading this and have already had your baby and that's fine, this is also for you. But when I was pregnant the first time, I didn't do anything to prepare for my breastfeeding journey – I didn't research, I didn't buy a book, I was also not given any information from healthcare professionals. Essentially, I went into it completely blind. I now know how important it is to prepare yourself. Don't get me wrong, I was able to breastfeed my eldest for 19 months through sheer determination, but I came across a lot of hurdles at the time and I did not know what to do or what to expect. If I had known what I know now when I first ever breastfed, I honestly believe and know our breastfeeding journey would have run a lot smoother, especially in the early days.

I spent my first pregnancy getting obsessed with learning about hypnobirthing, writing the strictest birthing plan known to man, but not bothering to do much research on breastfeeding. Honestly, I kick myself now, because I realise how naive I was back then. I had a huge lack of knowledge and not doing any kind of research just goes to prove that.

If you are reading this and thinking you want to give breastfeeding a go, I hope by the end of this book you will be thinking, *I know I can breastfeed my baby*. And you are then able to make the decision you feel is right for you and your baby or babies. After all, breastfeeding is 90 per cent determination and 10 per cent milk – mindset plays a huge part, too.

When I wanted to breastfeed the twins, I started my pregnancy with zero knowledge or research and I said to myself and my family in the beginning, 'OK, maybe I can combi-feed and at least I can breastfeed a little bit.' At the end of my pregnancy, after A LOT of research and fuelling my brain with knowledge, in my mind I would often tell myself, *I know 100 per cent I can breastfeed twins, my body is made to do this. I made two babies in my womb at the same time, of course my body can feed two babies too*. In my mind, there was no other option, I didn't have any bottles or formula as a 'just in case'! I was going to breastfeed and that was all there was to it. Out of those two attitudes, the one that wanted to give it a go but didn't know much compared to the 'We are doing this, I can do this', I know which one will go on to more than likely have a successful breastfeeding journey and which may come up against more hurdles. So, let's get you prepared – hopefully, before your baby arrives – so you can confidently enjoy a successful breastfeeding journey and maybe even fall in love with it, just like I did. Let me start by telling you to expect the unexpected!

Get yourself on the internet

Find your own little network of support. The first thing I would recommend to any mum wanting to breastfeed is to join a Breastfeeding Facebook support group. I cannot stress enough how much this will help you. This was the best thing I did for my breastfeeding journey second time around with the twins. The one I joined was particularly aimed at mums of twins and triplets wanting to breastfeed, but there are also a lot of other Facebook groups aimed at mums with singleton babies (one baby). Make sure the admins of your chosen group have some training in breastfeeding. You want to make sure their support is also evidence-based.

The support and knowledge from mums and breast-feeding specialists in these groups is second to none; just having that support, even via the internet, made me feel so confident and inspired. I learnt so much by reading all of the questions mums were asking and the answers that were given by other mums that had gone through it, plus the breastfeeding consultants which appeared on my timeline daily. When you are scrolling through your feed, you will constantly soak up knowledge and infor-mation. I learned things I hadn't even thought about and then put them to good use once my babies had arrived.

There are a lot of website-based forums where you can build up a network and connection, but always be mindful on the internet of the information you are receiving. If everyone is saying the same thing, you know that you are probably receiving good advice, plus if the admins are lactation consultants, they can tell you if they don't think you have received the correct or right amount of knowledge. Also, there are great Instagram pages dedicated to breastfeeding (*see also* Support, pages 249–53). They might be breastfeeding consultants, or breastfeeding charities, but once again, it's a great thing to see as you are scrolling through your timeline.

Get your support network around you, in the flesh

As I've said, one battle I had to overcome in both of my pregnancies was the negative opinions from other people (some family members) telling me I shouldn't breastfeed. (I know, it's craziness, there are literally not enough words to tell you how much this baffles me.) I politely in the beginning, and quite bluntly by the end, let everyone know how I wanted to feed MY children and all I asked was for their support in my decision. If you come up against negativity from people you know, love and trust, or even health professionals, it can feel upsetting and to be totally honest with you, I think it's disrespectful. When it comes to negativity for your choice with breastfeeding, it's important to stand up for yourself and let people know that this is not what you want to hear.

Luckily, the closest family members to me and all of my friends were nothing but supportive, even friends who had never breastfed before were so encouraging when it came to my wishes. These are the people you want to surround yourself with and speak about your breastfeeding to. It's a shame it has to be that way, but speaking about your goals or problems to someone who has been negative in the past about your breast-feeding may discourage you and if you're having a bad day, they are not the people that will be able to help the situation – you want a driving force of encourage-ment behind you.

Speak with your midwife

Let your midwife know your wishes and hopefully you will have a great one who can steer you in the right direction. They should be able to recommend a class for you in your area, which covers breastfeeding, but bear in mind it really is still not enough information, so it's still important to do more than just that. Find out where your local breastfeeding groups are and get the number of your nearest lactation consultant (the Lactation Consultants of Great Britain website – www .lcgb.org – is a good place to start) if the midwife isn't forthcoming with that information. Speak to your health visitor as they will know of volunteers who can help and support mums. It will really help you before your baby comes to find out where is best to turn to should you have any breastfeeding problems. If you are struggling and have a newborn baby, you don't want to just start researching for local lactation consultants or drop-in centres. Of course it's never too late, but ideally, it would be great to be prepared so if you do need to see someone for help, or maybe just have some questions you would like answered, then you are one step ahead as you know where to turn to straight away.

Research, research, research

Buy books, research on the internet. Join the Facebook groups, ask questions there. The more questions you ask, the more answers you get! Pick up leaflets from the hospital. Speak to friends who may have breastfed – even if they weren't able to breastfeed successfully, they will be able to let you know their struggles, what they found the hardest, and then you can make sure you have looked into how to overcome those problems to hopefully be able to have your own successful breastfeeding journey. Make sure you do not let anyone put you off, people love to tell horror stories and make things so much worse than they may have been. Take them in, research how to get over problems so if they do arise on your breastfeeding journey, you are already well equipped to handle the situation!

Get positive

You may have breastfed before and maybe it didn't get off to the best start. Do not let that put you off breast-feeding again. I know many women who struggled the first time, who then went on to successfully breastfeed their second, third, fourth children. Do not let any previous journeys put you off, or anyone else's stories. With any negative stories you may have heard or read, find out how that situation could have had a more positive outcome so that you are one step ahead.

Change your mindset: remember, your body was designed to do this. Making a baby and being pregnant are a lot harder for your body to do than producing milk, so do not doubt your capability. Write down positive breastfeeding affirmations and stick them around your bedroom (there are lots throughout this book), or even listen to positive breastfeeding meditation on YouTube. This is a great way to tap into your subconscious and if you are feeling worried and overloaded with doubt, taking five minutes to relax, clear your mind and listen to positivity only does you good. If you are feeling negative before you have even started your breastfeeding journey, there are many ways to change your mindset. And if you are feeling positive then you have gotten over the first hurdle!

Mentally prepare yourself

It's important to remember that just because breastfeeding is 'natural' doesn't mean it will be easy. If you love getting your beauty sleep, that's about to come to an end. But remember, it's not forever. Whether you choose to breastfeed, express, combi-feed or formula feed, your baby is going to want milk around the clock, and the first six weeks especially will feel very monotonous and I cannot express enough how tired you will feel. Knowing this can at the very least prepare you even just a little bit: it's a short period of time and, as I said, will not last forever.

This is going to sound so bizarre but sometimes I do miss waking up in the night for feeding. It's so peaceful and it's just you and your baby having one-on-one bonding time. It feels like the rest of the world is asleep and you are having your own little moment. When I was waking up through the night with all of my girls, something I told myself constantly was, 'I will miss this one day', because if you can see past the exhaustion it really is so special. I know I will never get those moments again in my life and they are so precious even when you are absolutely bloody exhausted!

Although breastfeeding is one of the most natural things in the world, it doesn't always come naturally to new mums – and that's completely normal. I have experienced so many mums saying no one tells you how unnatural it feels in the beginning and that it made them feel like they had failed. Well, please know that you haven't. I would say the majority of mums do not feel they took to breastfeeding like a duck to water. Breastfeeding is like learning to ride a bike, practice makes perfect, and perseverance will get you there.

Expect the early days to take up a lot of time while you are mastering this new skill. With the twins, I knew how crucial the first six weeks were. I made minimal plans and the only dates in my diary were skin-to-skin with my girls, in bed, with lots of boxsets, food and drink. I had one shot to get it right and put in the groundwork before it eased up and it wasn't so full-time.

IT IS SO MUCH HARDER
THAN YOU THINK, BUT
ONCE YOU CRACK IT, IT
IS EVEN MORE AMAZING
THAN YOU EVER THOUGHT
IT WOULD BE.

2

So, You've Just Given Birth

So, you've just given birth to your beautiful baby, what next? In an ideal, fairly straightforward scenario, your baby will be placed straight onto you for some skin-to-skin contact. The benefits for baby and Mum having skin-to-skin at this time are incredible. It has been scientifically proven to be one of the best things you can do and can really help to kickstart your breastfeeding journey[1]. Skin-to-skin also regulates baby's temperature, heart rate, breathing and increases blood glucose levels. I made it known to my husband and midwife when I was in labour with my first child that I wanted one hour of skin-to-skin to initiate breastfeeding and get to study this little human I had created and kept safe in my womb for nine months.

The Golden First Hour

Uninterrupted skin-to-skin the moment your baby is born is obviously not always possible due to complications that can arise during your labour and birth. If you don't

---

[1] Laleche.org.uk/whats-big-deal-skin-skin/

get to experience this 'Golden Hour' because there are many reasons why you might not be able to, all probably reasons beyond your control, then when you do hold your baby for the first time it will be just as special and amazing. Soak it all in, that newborn bubble is pretty special, no matter when you get to cuddle for the first time. Do not be too hard on yourself after you have just delivered your baby into the world.

If you have a pretty straightforward birth and a healthy baby then there is no reason why you shouldn't be able to experience this. Your baby does not need to be rushed off to be cleaned and weighed – that can wait, I promise! This is your time now and no one can take that away from you.

You've waited for this moment, very patiently, for nine months. Let's face it, that last month feels like a year on its own. Those first few minutes when your baby is placed on your chest are the most magical. We all hear about Mum and baby bonding, but there is so much research that proves just how amazing it is for the two of you to have your uninterrupted skin-to-skin in the first hour of your baby's life. Your baby wants to come into this world feeling safe and warm, put straight onto you, feeling your warmth, taking in your smell . . . They do not want to be rushed off, cleaned and placed on cold scales the moment they have arrived. It's important to try and make the transition as smoothly and comfortably as possible; this will have more benefits for you and your baby and it also helps to kickstart your breastfeeding journey.

If for whatever reason you yourself cannot do skin-to-skin, then it's a great opportunity for your partner to be able to do this.

Benefits of skin-to-skin

- Regulates baby's heart rate and breathing
- Regulates temperature
- Stimulates the hormone to help breastfeeding
- Improves breast milk production
- Helps regulate baby's blood sugar
- Promotes growth
- Keeps baby warm
- Calms baby so they are less likely to be distressed or cry
- Increases levels of love and nurturing for Mum
- Protects delayed cord clamping.
- Strengthens the immune system from Mum's bacteria

Breast Crawl

There is something called 'breast crawl', which is when your baby is placed on your abdomen and a specific part of the baby's brain is stimulated, and they crawl to their mum's breast and are able to feed on their own. Seriously, how crazy and magical is that? Search 'Breast Crawl' on YouTube – there are some amazing videos where you can see a baby doing this.

Your baby uses their hands, limbs and the senses of sight, smell and sound to 'get to know' their mum. You may be wondering why your nipples got darker and larger in your pregnancy. It is for this reason: to help your baby find your nipple and latch correctly. (If you're wondering if this happened to me, then yes, yes, it did – I thought this was how they would always be, but they slowly returned to how they were pre-pregnancy.)

As your baby reaches your breasts and touches them with their palms and hands, you will experience a surge of oxytocin, the love hormone. Not only will you experience this, so too will your child. I was lucky enough to experience this with Dakota, my eldest, and it really was truly magical and so fascinating to watch. Your tiny little baby that has just come into the world has the ability to crawl up your body, find your breasts and latch on all by themselves. Remember, all babies are different: some take longer than others, you may have had no interventions, or you may have had some form of pain relief, which can affect how alert your baby is.

Before I had children, I watched videos online, 'How to Latch Your Baby', and for some reason, they made me feel anxious and I started to doubt my ability to do it. I don't particularly like my nipples being touched, so the thought of latching a baby onto them made me feel a little bit uncomfortable, so I pushed these thoughts to the back of my head and didn't watch any more videos online, which was narrow-minded of me. When I gave birth to my eldest, she latched onto me herself within half an hour of giving birth, so she took that first time out of my hands and did it all herself.

I thought that would be it, it was much easier than expected and we had cracked it, but it wasn't that easy. After a week or so of breastfeeding, my nipples cracked and it became very painful to feed. I don't want to downplay this to you, but I don't want to put you off either, so please know this doesn't happen to every mum and it didn't happen to me when I had the twins, just with Dakota. The pain was excruciating and was likely to do with a shallow latch – many others find they have sore nipples to begin with. Seeking support early is the key to avoiding cracked, painful nipples! But I carried on, became better at achieving a deeper latch as my baby grew, my nipples got used to the feeding and I had a successful breastfeeding journey.

FUN FACT

Breast milk changes due to biological sex
As the composition of breast milk is completely tailored to your baby's needs, it's no surprise that your breast milk changes composition when feeding boys or girls. Milk produced by mothers of baby boys contains more fat and protein, while milk produced by mothers of baby girls contains higher levels of calcium.[2] Interesting stuff, hey?

[2] www.imedpub.com/articles/biochemical-differences-in-human-breastmilk-contents-according-to-infants-gender.php?aid=23183

COMFORT, LOVE,
NUTRITION, SERVED
ON DEMAND.

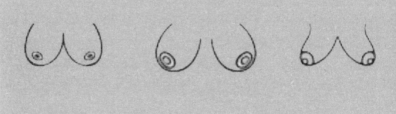

PART 2

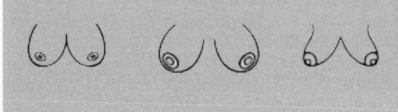

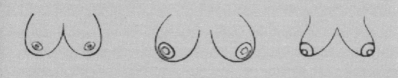

MILKING IT

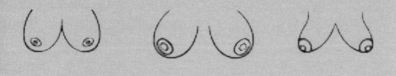

3

Understanding Milk Production

I think it's absolutely crucial for every breastfeeding mum to know and understand how her body makes milk and how her supply works. This information will give you confidence in your ability to feed your baby but it will also help you to not doubt your milk supply. Plus, if you are anything like me, you will find this really interesting and be amazed by how our bodies work.

Your breast milk production works on a supply and demand system. Someone once told me that your breast milk supply works like a factory and not a warehouse – your breasts will ALWAYS have milk. The more milk you remove from your breasts, the more milk your body will produce – it really is that simple.

Your body is producing milk all the time, around the clock: before you feed, when you are feeding and after you have fed. Your breasts will work like a tap, the milk will always be flowing and they are never really empty. It's important you don't wait for your boobs to 'fill up' with milk before another feed, as waiting for longer periods of time actually signals to your breasts you need less milk, which in turn means your body will produce less milk. The more you feed your baby, the more milk your body produces. The milk will always be there ready and waiting for your child, as and when they need it.

The structure of the breast

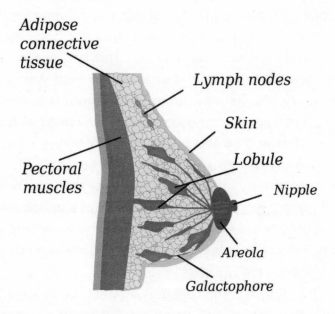

Quite often when mums start to doubt their milk supply, they might add formula top-ups. If you want to continue breastfeeding your baby exclusively then supplementing with formula will actually reduce your milk supply, as you will be missing out on an opportunity to remove more milk from your breasts. Remember, the more milk you remove, the more milk your body will produce. The less you feed, the less milk your body will make. Sometimes, if a baby has not been feeding well, your milk supply can take a little time to catch up, and so this is where a little formula can be useful.

Misconceptions of low milk supply

Babies feed round the clock, and the average baby feeds around 11 times in 24 hours. It's important to remember they also breastfeed for comfort, to feel close to you, not just because they are hungry. Plus, you never really know how much milk they are getting at each feed. The following are all issues that are perfectly normal:

1. Wanting to feed constantly – This is known as 'cluster feeding'. When this happens, it is normally because babies are going through a growth spurt or developmental leaps. Growth spurts normally last two to three days but can last up to a week.
2. Baby waking through the night – Night feeds are so important for your milk supply, and in order for your baby to grow, they need to feed. They have small tummies that need filling regularly!
3. Long or short feeds – Some babies feed quickly, others do not. The older they get, the more efficient they become at feeding so may feed a lot quicker, but the next day they may feed for longer, they may feel unwell or they may feed purely because they want

to be close to you. Babies feed for more reasons than being hungry.

4. Your baby will feed from a bottle even after a feed from the breast – Babies are born with a sucking reflex (those born before 36 weeks will still be developing). This is an involuntary reflex, so of course even if your baby is full from your breast, they will still drink from a bottle even if they do not feel hungry.

5. When you use a breast pump, and you feel that you aren't expressing much breast milk – A lot of mums worry that when they pump and they aren't getting a lot of milk, that this means they have a low milk supply, but it's important to know that how much you pump is actually no indication of your milk supply, so please do not let this put you off and make you worry. A plastic pump is nowhere near as effective at removing milk as your baby. When your baby feeds from you, not only are they more efficient at removing milk but they also contribute to the hormones which help your milk to flow, and these same hormones are not released when using a pump.

6. Your boobs aren't leaking and are soft – Some women just do not ever leak and if you have leaked before and have been feeding for a few weeks then this is actually a good sign. When your boobs stop leaking, this is a sign that your breasts are regulating the correct amount of milk, know your baby's feeding pattern and have adjusted accordingly. However, some

women leak throughout their breastfeeding journey, even once milk supply has regulated.

7. You have small boobs – Size is no indication of milk supply. I have also heard of women put off trying breastfeeding as they do not have big boobs and they think they wouldn't be able to breastfeed for this reason. The size of breasts is down to the fatty tissues that do not have anything to do with producing milk. Sometimes smaller boobs may produce more milk than larger ones and vice versa.

These are the signs that you may have a low milk supply:

1. Poor weight gain – All babies lose weight after they are born, it is normal for them to lose around 6 per cent of their birth weight and some up to 10 per cent in the first few days of their life. If you go over the 10 per cent, this is normally when the midwife or health visitor will suggest formula top-ups. But it is so very important to take into consideration how your labour went too. Were you on a drip, did you have a C-section? These may contribute to the weight of your baby when they are born, so the weight loss may be higher than usual. Your baby will normally start to gain weight around days 4 to 6 and will normally regain their birth weight around ten to 14 days later. If they were premature or unwell, then it may take a little longer to get back to their birth weight. You should be supported to pump your milk to give

to your baby and should be signposted to breast-feeding support to find out why your baby has lost too much weight. There is often a simple solution (like improving latch, not limiting feeds, baby being sleepy etc.).

2. Not enough dirty or wet nappies – If you are worried about your milk supply, this is a great way for you to know whether your baby is getting enough milk. Before there were bottles and formula, mums did not know how much milk their breasts stored and would simply know they were doing well by their baby's nappy output. The first day of your baby's life, expect one wet nappy, day two expect two, day three expect three, up until day six – where you can expect at least six wet nappies a day from then onwards. On day one expect to see at least one meconium poo, and then at least two to three poos a day from then on. Some babies may poo more than this and that's fine, don't worry about too much poo!

As your milk comes in, around days 3 to 6, you should be seeing about three dirty nappies and six to eight wet nappies over a 24-hour period. Once they reach four to six weeks of age, they could poo every day, more than once a day, and it's not unusual for babies that are exclusively breastfed to go up to ten days or even two weeks without pooing. With breast milk, there is normally very little waste left for your baby to poo, so the first month of their life, when you are probably worrying the most about your milk supply, the clear indication will be what is going into your baby's nappies.

Some women may have a genuine low milk supply due to medical issues and they may or may not be aware of this before the baby arrives. Here are some causes:

1. Previous breast surgery or trauma – Whether you had breast surgery for medical or cosmetic reasons, there may be some damage to your milk ducts. This doesn't mean you won't be able to breastfeed, but it is something important to be aware of as it may limit the amount of milk you are able to produce. I personally know a lot of women who have had breast surgery, cosmetically and medically, and have been able to breastfeed.

2. Hormonal problems – You may have polycystic ovaries, low or high thyroid, diabetes or other hormonal disorders. These can sometimes cause low milk supply as they may not be able to efficiently send hormonal signals to your breasts to supply milk.

3. Mammary hypoplasia – A very uncommon condition, also known as insufficient glandular tissue (IGT), which means during adolescence you would not have developed enough mammary tissue. Signs you have this include widely spaced boobs, very small or tubular shaped boobs, areolas that look swollen or puffy, and most importantly, you have no breast changes in pregnancy.

4. Traumatic Birth – Blood loss during or after labour, leading to anaemia or having a retained placenta, can delay your milk coming in. The hormone oxytocin, which is vital to milk production, travels through the blood so it makes sense that there may be a delay.

For the above reasons, I would highly recommend finding a lactation consultant (*see also* Support, pages 250–51) and speaking with your doctor before you give birth. Talk through any concerns and they will be able to give you the best advice to help with your milk supply. Please know that the above reasons do not mean you will not be able to breastfeed. They may affect your supply, they may not, you might be able to breastfeed exclusively, you may have to combi-feed.

Of course, you might actually have low milk supply that is not down to health or medical reasons. If this is more like the issue rather than any of the above then I'm confident that you can increase your chances of upping your supply. Here are some reasons why your milk supply may be low:

1. Taking certain medications, like decongestants and some contraceptives, is not recommended while breastfeeding as they may substantially decrease your milk supply. Most medications are safe to take whilst breastfeeding but if you are not sure or have been told a medication is not safe, contact the

Breastfeeding Network's 'Drugs in Breastmilk' website or Facebook page to get advice.

2. Incorrect latching – A shallow latch can mean the feed is less efficient and so milk supply is not stimulated as well. Your baby may have something like tongue-tie (*see also* pages 117–18) and this is something that can be rectified if you see your doctor or a lactation consultant.

3. Scheduled feeding or using a dummy – These will interfere with the supply and demand process and you may miss feeding cues from your baby. It's important to feed every time your baby shows feeding cues. Responsive feeding, commonly referred to as feeding on demand, normally makes feeding calmer, ensures a baby feels secure and optimises milk supply and more efficient.

4. Topping up with formula – As stated at the beginning of this chapter, not removing milk from your body means you don't send as many signals to your body to produce it. But sometimes it is necessary if your baby is not feeding well and you are suddenly struggling to produce more. The good news is, with good breastfeeding support, your baby can learn to feed more efficiently and you can be supported to increase your supply. Often mums can move back to breastfeeding exclusively if they wish.

5. Not feeding at night – There are lots of books on how to get your babies to sleep longer through the night,

but usually they don't mention how not breastfeeding through the night can damage your milk supply. There is more prolactin (the hormone that signals the breasts to make milk) during night feeds, so not missing these times is so important in keeping your supply up.

6. Nipple shields – Now, I know these can be lifesavers! Personally, they really helped to latch my girls on in the early days. But they can sometimes hinder your milk supply as they may reduce the stimulation to your nipple, which in return interferes with the supply and demand process. It is best to use these under the supervision of a breastfeeding supporter. They can be very useful for babies born before 37 weeks, babies with tongue-tie, and those who are mostly bottle fed to encourage them back to the breast, but should be used with caution.

Increasing milk supply

1. The first thing I would suggest is to find a local lactation consultant (see also Support, 251). Make sure your lactation consultant has the International Board Certified Lactation Consultant (IBCLC) qualification. This will ensure they have the correct training. Not only will a lactation consultant give you the confidence to know your body and how it works, but they will also provide you with all the correct tools and information to help make your

journey possible. They can do an oral assessment and check if your baby is feeding efficiently, check your baby's latch or maybe change the position you are feeding in, and talk about normal baby behaviour. If you have started supplementing formula but would like to breastfeed exclusively, they should be able to put together a feeding plan to help up your milk supply.

2. Pump – This is something that really helped to increase my milk supply in the early days with the twins. After every feed, I would use a breast pump and at the start it seemed I was only pumping small amounts, but after a few days I really noticed a big difference. In the early days, you feed around eight to 12 times a day and I used to pump after each of these feeds. Don't get me wrong, it was time-consuming with twin babies and a three-year-old, but the only choice I wanted was to breastfeed, so I put in the groundwork at the beginning and it paid off as the twins were breastfed exclusively for over two years. It is important to use a hospital grade double pump if you are looking to pump more than just here and there (these can be hired or bought) and to do massage before and during the pumping session to increase the flow.

Something I have heard that is very effective but did not try out myself is power pumping. Pumping for one hour a day over three to four days can help your supply. It's meant to replicate when a baby cluster feeds (*see also* pages 67–75), so it's a bit like boot camp for breastfeeding! Below is a guide to how it works:

- Double pump for 20 minutes
- Rest for ten minutes
- Double pump for ten minutes
- Rest for ten minutes
- Double pump for ten minutes.

3. Breastfeed as frequently as possible. If you are worried about your supply, or your baby is having issues with their weight, then feed around every one and a half to two hours.
4. Alone time – Something that helped me was arranging a few days in a row of no visitors, so me and the girls could lay in bed, nursing to their hearts' content, with me pumping afterwards. This also encouraged lots of skin-to-skin, which is great for upping milk supply, too.
5. Stay hydrated (drink to thirst – bring water with you everywhere!), eat well and look after your mental health. People say, 'Happy mum, happy baby' and this also helps when it comes to your milk supply. If you can, take time out for you to be the healthiest version you can be. I know this is not always possible when you have a newborn baby to look after on top of everything else, but after every feed I always tried to drink 600ml (1 pint) water – something simple, but it was an easy way to remember to drink, as

often we forget to take care of ourselves. It is good to have someone to look after the mum so the mum can look after the baby.

FUN FACT

Breast milk composition changes
Breast milk is physically impossible to replicate as it is so unique, alive and changes throughout your breastfeeding journey. The composition of your breast milk does change to meet the specific needs of your baby at different times of day, and it can even change during one feed. In the summer when it is hotter, your milk will have an increase in water to make sure your baby remains hydrated without needing to intake water separately.[1]

---

[1] https://www.ncbi.nlm.nih.gov/pmc/articles/PMC3586783/

SHE BELIEVED SHE COULD, SO SHE DID.

4

Cluster Feeding

This has nothing to do with low milk supply, but when your baby is going through a stage of cluster feeding, it is one of the most common misconceptions women make for thinking they have a low milk supply. I've had a huge number of mums tell me their story: 'I wasn't ready to stop breastfeeding, but at six weeks my milk just dried up', 'I was so upset my body just ran out of milk at six weeks, the baby was starving'.

Every time I hear this, it breaks my heart. I just wish so much that they had had support from someone or somewhere with breastfeeding knowledge. As you've just read, if you have been breastfeeding successfully for six weeks, putting your baby to your boob at their hunger cues, they are having dirty and wet nappies and gaining weight, then your baby is not starving. Your body works based on supply and demand, so remember, it will stop producing milk if you stop demanding it. You can also re-lactate your breasts (*see also* Chapter 11, pages 121–24), so to just run out of milk when your baby has been feeding effectively for weeks does not seem right.

What is cluster feeding?

This is a very clever way for your baby to increase your milk supply ahead of a growth spurt, and is when your baby wants lots of short feeds. Your child has a natural instinct in them to effectively teach your body to make more milk. This does not mean they need more milk than your body can provide, so remember adding formula will send a signal to your body to release less milk.

Cluster feeding is very normal and although it can occur at any time of day, it is more common in the evening. Evening cluster feeding is not just about food, it is also for comfort and to help babies relax. If they have had a particularly busy day, lots of stimulation or an overload of visitors, you may notice that they are cluster feeding more. One evening while we were away on holiday as a family, I found it all a bit too much, so Lewis took the twins out for a walk in their pram so I could have a little breather and get ready for some more feeding. Your baby may be really fussing, going on your boob for a few minutes and then coming off, screaming and fussing, going back on again and so on. You might give them a feed and then they want to feed immediately after. If you do not know about cluster feeding, how are you supposed to know this is NORMAL?! I can totally understand why any mum would start to doubt their milk supply, but please let me tell you this IS normal. It is a very normal pattern for a lot of babies between 3 and 12 weeks, so don't panic.

But remember, it's not forever. I knew I had to get through this tough, relentless stage to reach the amazing, rewarding part that more than made up for it.

How can cluster feeding make you feel?

I remember the cluster-feeding days oh so well – they were relentless! I would lay one of the twins down and then they would want more. I felt exhausted and at times extremely frustrated. It's crap at the time and I'm pretty certain I cried my way through one of our cluster-feeding phases as you feel that it's all completely on you. I would feel pissed off at my husband – I knew he couldn't do anything about it! It made me anxious for the afternoons to start because I knew what I was going to be faced with. Did I have times when I wanted to quit? Hell, yes, I did! I often doubted myself, not my milk supply but my own capabilities. Could I keep this up with not one baby but TWO tiny demanding mouths? I knew in the back of my mind, and would continuously tell myself, *This is not forever*. Someone once told me, which has never left me, 'Do not give up on a bad day, as tomorrow could be your best day.' It's really true.

Please do not feel like you're failing, or that you're alone in these tough stages. I guarantee every mum who has breastfed will have gone through these cluster-feeding periods and experienced exactly what you are. This is why a lot of people doubt their supply, as they feel like their boobs are empty. Remember, your breasts NEVER empty, the milk river is constantly flowing and the feeling in your breasts is zero indication of your supply. Even in the midst of a feeding frenzy there is research to suggest that your breasts will still have 25 per cent capacity of milk in them.

If you have joined a Facebook support group and are experiencing cluster feeding, this might be a great time to write your first post as I'm sure the support and encouragement you will get from others that have experienced this stage and got through it will put your mind at rest, reassure and inspire you. YOU GOT THIS!

Things to remember and note:

- Are they gaining weight?
- Are they having wet nappies? (remember, dirty nappies can only be relied upon in the first month or so)
- Are they alert?

If your answer is 'yes' to these and you do not have any medical or health-related reasons for low milk supply, and the only reason you doubt your supply is due to your baby feeding a lot and maybe not seeming satisfied, then the first thing that would come to mind is cluster feeding. To be able to tackle this in your head, I think it's very important to know when cluster feeding is more likely to arise because then straight away, you are already one step ahead of the game.

Growth spurts

This is more than likely the main reason why your baby may be cluster feeding, as well as developmental leaps. It's important to take your baby's lead and keep feeding when they want and need it, even if you think they don't. This is how we have fed babies for thousands of years, so you can trust the system.

The biggest growth spurt is at six weeks, give or take a week. This is the toughest growth spurt of them all and why I mentioned before that mums often say at six weeks, their milk dried up. This seems to me the most typical time women doubt their milk supply.

Growth spurts can really come at any time, although there are the key common ones that most mums seem to experience:

- Around two to three weeks
- The BIG one at six to eight weeks
- Twelve weeks
- Four months
- Six months
- Nine months.

But it's important to remember that just like you and I, babies are all programmed differently and these numbers are just a guide. A mum contacted me at seven weeks, saying her supply had definitely run out, as she could feed for hours and then ten minutes later, her baby wanted to feed again. I asked the questions, is your baby gaining weight? Are they alert? Do they have wet nappies? Yes, yes, and yes. She said her baby definitely didn't have a six-week growth spurt, so maybe they didn't tell her body to up her milk supply and it just ran out. This is highly unlikely to have happened. I asked her to keep at it for a few more days, a week maximum, and to see if he went back to feeding normally. And of course, what do you know, he did. (There is a growth spurt normally documented between six to eight weeks.) So what I'm saying here is babies do not read calendars, they don't just think, *I'm six weeks today, I'm going to up my mum's milk supply*. It's an instinct built within them, so your growth spurts might not be bang to the day, they could happen a week before or a week after. It may seem like you have a low milk supply but it's highly unlikely you do, so remind yourself about wet nappies and weight gain.

The only thing that got me through the growth spurts was knowing in advance when they were likely to happen so I was fully prepared for it, and also knowing that they normally only last two to three days, or sometimes up to a week.

Reasons why babies breastfeed

You now know how milk production works and I have explained the reasons why you might think you have low milk supply, but breast milk is so much more than just food. Your baby will also want to feed for emotional reasons. Just to give you a little extra confidence about your breast milk and your body, and also because this is so bloody interesting, here are some reasons why your baby wants milk!

1. The most obvious: they are hungry or thirsty.
2. Your baby is tired: breast milk contains melatonin, a sleep-inducing hormone.
3. They may be coming down with a bug: if babies have been exposed to an illness, their saliva will signal to your body to get your breast milk to produce antibodies to help fight against the illness they have been exposed to.
4. Your baby may be feeling scared: they know you, your smell and your comfort. You make them feel safe, so breastfeeding is a perfect way for them to feel reassured.
5. They may be in pain: your own breast milk is a good analgesic for your baby. Not only does your baby gain comfort from suckling on your breast, expressed breast milk can help relieve pain in babies.
6. Your baby may be feeling cold: the warmth from your snuggling while breastfeeding can warm them.
7. Maybe they have been overstimulated and need to relax and calm down.
8. This is only relevant if you are feeding multiples, or an older sibling, but every time I fed one twin, the

other twin would want to breastfeed, the only reason being because their sibling was.

9. They are going through a growth spurt and have a natural instinct to up your milk supply.
10. They may just want to feel comforted: breastfeeding is known to release the 'love hormone' oxytocin, not only in your baby but also in yourself. This will make you feel calm and close to one another.
11. Simply because they love you and want to feel close to you.

You cannot overfeed your baby, the answer to most things for your breastfed child is to breastfeed. When in doubt, whip it out!

Can you experience oversupply?

I know you may be reading this and thinking, what's wrong with having oversupply, surely that's great? If I have lots of milk for my baby, what's the problem?

Obviously, it's great that your baby is gaining weight and thriving, but I have spoken with a few mums who struggled in the early days due to their oversupply. If your breasts are producing more milk than your baby actually needs, this could make your breasts feel rather uncomfortable. It can be distressing for your baby and of course you as well.

There are a few signs why you may think you have oversupply, but it can be hard to tell, as some of the signs could be for something else and some can also be completely normal. If you are worrying in the first six weeks or so, your body is regulating your breast milk and it is absolutely crucial that you do not try and drop your milk supply at this time. I would only advise you doing so once it has been confirmed by a breastfeeding counsellor or certified consultant you have oversupply.

Signs of oversupply include: your milk may flow (spray) out too fast, which in turn might mean your baby swallows a lot of air as well as your milk, making them agitated and very windy; your breasts may feel like they are always full and hard; often your breasts become easily engorged. As always, if you are in doubt, contact a breastfeeding counsellor or consultant.

DON'T CRY OVER SPILT MILK, UNLESS IT'S BREAST MILK – IN WHICH CASE, CRY A LOT!

5

Latching

Let me talk you through latching so you can learn how to do it correctly and what to do to help you if your nipples become sore. I had no idea about latching after having my first child, and our latch in the early days was not correct – it was too shallow, which led to me being in a lot of discomfort.

The most important part of any successful breastfeeding journey is the latch. I think there is a misconception that babies just suck on your nipple like a straw, but this is not correct. I know this is what I certainly thought!

When you are in hospital, and intending on breastfeeding, hopefully you will have a midwife with good knowledge and they can check your latch and advise you, or maybe your hospital will have a breastfeeding consultant who can help you. If no one comes round, then please make sure you ask to see someone to check they are happy with how your baby is latching, so by the time you and your baby are discharged from hospital, you can leave feeling confident of your latch.

You cannot always bank on this, though. The breastfeeding consultants at my hospital did not work weekends, so when I gave birth to twins on a Friday evening,

I didn't have anyone from the breastfeeding team able to check the girls' latches and we were discharged on the Monday afternoon. So, it's important to know the facts yourself; learn what you need to know, this will give you some confidence to be one step ahead:

1. First things first, get yourself in a comfortable position. Bring your baby to you and remember, don't bend down to your baby, lift them to you and where your breasts are. This will make you more comfortable and also affects your baby's position.
2. Hold your baby close to you to encourage them to try and latch themselves. This is not always possible, but it's good to try.
3. Place your index finger and thumb behind your baby's ears so your palm is behind their neck. This way you are supporting them without holding their head. (It's good for your baby to be able to move their head back before they latch on, chin first.)
4. Start with your baby's nose in line with your nipple, brush their top lip with your nipple to encourage them to open wide and route.
5. Make sure your baby's jaw is wide open, enough to get a good mouthful of areola and not just your nipple.
6. If your baby has a small mouth, you might want to help by moving your hands further back from your areola – about two to three inches, make a C shape with your fingers and thumb if your baby is on their back, or a U shape if they are more on their side.

This really helped when my twins were born as they were five weeks early and didn't have the biggest mouths.

Signs of a good latch:

1. Baby's chin is touching your breast.
2. You should hear deep sucks and your baby swallowing. Your baby should not be clicking.
3. Deep jaw movement, ears wiggle and cheeks are rounded.
4. There is a gap between baby's nose and the breast.
5. Once your baby has finished feeding, your nipple is not misshapen.
6. Your baby is content after their feed – either they finish feeding themselves or nod off.

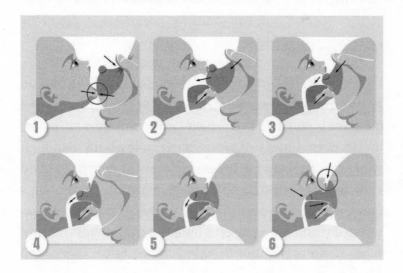

It is always good to watch videos online, so you can see first-hand, in action, what you need to be doing. Global Health Media has great videos on this – search 'attaching your baby at the breast' on their website.

If you have any concerns about your latch, then please get some face-to-face support; your midwife, health visitor or breastfeeding consultants are great people to reach out to, so they can check for you. If your baby isn't latching correctly, it can be painful but can also hinder your milk supply as your baby will not be feeding as efficiently. It's so important to get this first part correct to help your breastfeeding journey get off to a good start. If you are struggling with latching, please do not fear: help is available. I struggled with latching Dakota, my eldest, and the twins too, but following advice, we were still able to have a successful breastfeeding journey.

Your first feed

I remember the first time my eldest daughter latched on and knowing I was breastfeeding. It was one of the most overwhelming feelings I have ever experienced in my life to date. I had just given birth to my baby and now we were connected in a very different way to how I had ever been connected to anyone. High on hormones, I was the proudest person in the world! The oxytocin was flying around my body and I was on the biggest natural high. I also remember thinking that it felt so alien and wondering if breastfeeding would always feel strange to me – it didn't and it soon became normal in an amazing way.

As I told you earlier, I didn't get this same experience with my twins. Twin 1 (Tatum) was taken away after I gave birth to her as I then had to give birth to her sister, Twin 2 (Blakely, through an emergency C-section. While I was being stitched up, the midwife asked if I would like to see Twin 2 as I hadn't met her and my reply was 'I need to breastfeed her'! I just had this overwhelming urge to try and regain a connection as I disconnected myself the moment I knew I was to have an emergency C-section. She was so tiny and my nipple seemed so huge compared to her mouth, but we persevered and she latched on. I don't remember the first time feeding Twin 1, it was more than likely when I was in recovery and I was being physically milked by a midwife I had never met, but that's a whole different story . . .

What I'm trying to say is both my experiences of my first breastfeed, that 'Golden Hour', were completely different, but I was still able to go on and successfully breastfeed all three of my children. I feel like this is an important thing to mention as you might read all the ideal scenarios after you give birth, all of the amazing benefits of the one-hour skin-to-skin, but what if you don't get that time? Everyone's journey is different, and if you have chosen to breastfeed, your experiences will be different, so try not to panic and immediately start comparing yourself to everyone else.

TRUST YOUR BODY.

6

Feeding Cues

So, you've had your first feed, what next? Basically, you repeat that first feed around the clock when your baby wants to feed. They sleep a lot in the early days so it's important that you don't let them go any longer than three hours from the start of each feed – the maximum you should let your baby go without a feed. Roughly, in a 24-hour period, the minimum your baby should feed is eight to 12 times. Most babies like to feed far more frequently – on average, a baby feeds 11 times in 24 hours. But remember, each child is different – they may feed for 45 minutes and then want to feed again 30 minutes later, or they might feed for 30 minutes and then not want another feed for two hours. There is not a set routine when it comes to breastfeeding, it's just important to follow your baby's lead.

It's essential to follow your baby's feeding cues and if you're not sure if they're hungry, just feed. Once again, when in doubt, whip it out! Don't worry about missing feeding cues because your baby won't give up and you will soon know about it . . .!

Early feeding cues

- Stirring
- Mouth opening
- Licking lips
- Turning head (aka rooting), looking around for your nipple

Mid-cues

- Stretching
- More physical movement
- Hands to mouth (after six to eight weeks, babies have more control and like to explore, so this will not count as a feeding cue as they get older)

Late cutes

- Crying
- Agitated body

Your baby will latch and feed a lot better if you catch their early feeding cues as opposed to when they are screaming and very agitated, of course.

Your first feed after a C-section

There are many reasons you might have to have a C-section, whether it is planned or an emergency. All being well, there is no reason why you can't experience the same as someone having a vaginal birth with regards to the first feed and the Golden Hour. And if there is a reason why you cannot, then once again, your partner or birthing partner can step in, or you can have it later in recovery. Most hospitals are set up to offer immediate skin-to- skin after a caesarean. You can write it in your birth plan and ask for it when you are being prepared for the operation. It can be more difficult in the early days of breastfeeding – you will probably find it harder to find a comfortable position and the use of an epidural or IV fluids can make your baby sleepier. But as long as you keep putting your baby to the breast for feeds frequently, or if that's not possible then pumping frequently, your body will get the signal and there is no reason you won't be able to enjoy a wonderful breastfeeding journey.

If you are having a planned C-section, it's a great idea to speak with your midwife and consultant and let them know your wishes for breastfeeding, and that if everything is medically OK with you and your baby, you would like immediate skin-to-skin and to try breastfeeding, even while in recovery. I breastfed when I was still on the operating table being stitched up, with the help of my midwife, who was thankfully amazing. I was lying flat so it was difficult, but with the help of an extra pair of hands, it was possible – I have the whole moment of that first feed on camera!

There may be a reason you have to have a general anaesthetic, and although this is rare, it does happen.

You may wake up and feel really groggy, or there might be a medical reason you cannot be with your baby in the first 12 hours. I would suggest you request a hospital pump and following advice, hand express colostrum in the first 48 hours, then move to the pump once your milk begins to come in, pumping every two hours so your body still gets that signal (*see also* pages 63–64).

While I'm talking about colostrum, if you are having a planned C-section you could speak with your midwife about harvesting your colostrum in your thirty-seventh week of pregnancy, or the week before a planned C-section. That way, if your milk is delayed, you will still have your milk as a backup, which will take a massive stress off you. Also, it is important to add, you should find out from your hospital how long they will store your milk for – make sure it is labelled with your full name and the date it was expressed. It might be a good idea not to bring all your milk to the hospital at one time in case your hospital doesn't store it for long. To store your colostrum at home, make sure the syringes are placed into a resealable bag. It can be kept in your freezer for up to three months, or in your fridge for up to five days.

IT IS OK AND NORMAL
IF MY BABY FEEDS
FREQUENTLY.

7

Breastfeeding Positions

I remember when I was pregnant with Dakota, my eldest daughter, and I started researching breastfeeding positions. My mind was blown by the different positions in which you can breastfeed. It's important not to overthink things, it's all trial and error and what might work for one mum might not work for you. You may feel cack-handed at the start, or it could come completely naturally to you. There really is no right or wrong answer, but just remember, before you know it, you won't even be thinking of positions and it will all become second nature.

So, grab your snacks, drinks, cushions, breastfeeding pillow – whatever's going to make you feel most comfortable while feeding. Make sure you and your baby are comfortable, then half the battle is already won!

Different positions to try

Cradle hold/Cross cradle

If you were to picture a woman breastfeeding, it is probably this position that you will think of. You are sitting upright, with your baby cradled across your front, sup-porting them with the same arm as you are breastfeed-ing them from, for cradle, or the opposite arm for cross cradle. Make yourself comfortable on the sofa to have back support, and you can pop a cushion under your elbow too. Leaning back a little can make this more comfortable and your baby can drape over your tummy.

Laid-back breastfeeding

Lie back in a semi-reclined position, with your baby's face down on your stomach and their arms up around your boobs. This position fully supports your baby's body and helps to encourage a deep latch. Baby needs to be slightly under the breast and looking up at the nipple to get a deep latch.

Rugby/Clutch hold

If you were to imagine a rugby player running with the ball then you would picture them with a ball under their arm. This is exactly what the Rugby hold is – you have your baby tucked under the same side that you are breastfeeding from. Support baby's neck with fingers and thumbs behind the ears to give them support and also to guide them up on to your breast. This is great if you have had a C-section as you will have no pressure on your stitches. You will likely need a cushion or pillow to support your baby's body.

Side-lying positions

As it says on the tin! Lying down on your side, your baby facing you, stomach to stomach. Baby needs to be slightly lower than the breast, looking up at the nipple in order to get a deep latch. This position is great for night-time feeds as it is very relaxed and comfortable. It is also good to place some pillows behind your back for extra support.

Upright breastfeeding/Koala hold

This position is with you sitting upright and your baby straddled over your thigh, their legs either side. You can do this position for a newborn, but for me it was really efficient when my girls were older and able to support themselves, especially when I was breastfeeding in public. This is a great position for babies who are windy or who have reflux, too. You can also lean back a bit once baby is attached and feeding.

Breastfeeding positions for twins

Double Rugby hold

A great position for breastfeeding twins, and when I tandem fed my twins for the first time, this was the position we tried. It feels very alien in the early days, trying to latch two babies and feed, but it was not long before I was feeding them both and wasn't even

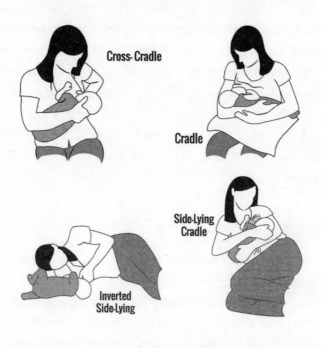

Cross-Cradle

Cradle

Side-Lying
Cradle

Inverted
Side-Lying

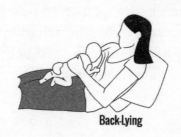

Back-Lying

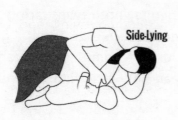

Side-Lying

Rugby

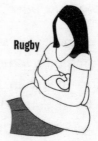

thinking about the positions. If you use a twin breast-feeding pillow that is a good height for your body shape, once they are latched on, you will have both hands free so you can go on your phone, have a drink of water, change the TV channel, maybe have some snacks. Your arms are pretty much free in this position and being able to tandem feed twins and still be able to use your hands is a great plus!

Rugby & Cradle

This one is a good position when if you are breastfeeding while out and about and might not have your twin cushion with you. One baby is in the Rugby hold, the other in the Cradle position, both your hands will be supporting your babies so you are less free. If you are round someone's house, you could pop some cushions under your elbows to make yourself more comfortable. You may need a cushion to help support the baby in Rugby hold, or alternatively if you're out you could use your changing bag or a rolled-up coat.

Double Laid-back

Recline and get comfy, then lay both twins facing you. Pop some pillows underneath each arm. This is a great position to get in for cluster-feeding sessions (and a good boxset on TV!). It can be a little fiddly to master this position, though.

Cross Cradle

Cradle each baby and have the same side arm as the breast they are latched onto supporting each child. This one is slightly more complicated, but as they get older, it will be easier to position them as they have more head control.

Double Upright

This is a great position for when your twins are older and can support their own heads. It was one of the positions I fed in when I tandem breastfed in public, each baby on one of my thighs and their legs straddled either side.

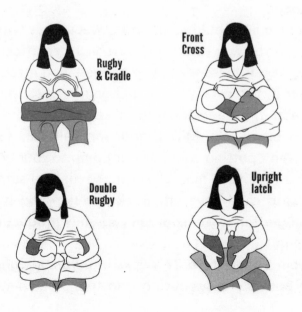

8

Your Baby's Stomach Size

A lot of women in the first few days after giving birth message me, panicking that their milk 'hasn't come in'. This is not something a new mum should be worrying about at this time. As long as your baby is latching correctly, and you are putting them to your breast regularly, you are fine. Only producing small amounts of colostrum, like 1ml, is very normal for the first few days.

Your milk should come in between days two and five, but the way you have given birth can affect how many days it takes for this to happen, and it can take longer if, for instance, you had pain medication during labour, a traumatic birth, C-section or more than 500ml blood loss. Milk production will only stop if you aren't putting your baby or pump to your breasts by the time your milk comes in, so making sure you and your child have lots of skin-to-skin and breast-feeding often will encourage your milk production to come in.

From about 16 to 22 weeks into your pregnancy, your body starts producing colostrum, (see page 99) a concentrated milk that is full of nutrients and disease-fighting antibodies. It provides your baby with everything they need in the first few days after giving birth when their stomach will only be able to hold roughly a teaspoon of colostrum. One teaspoon! Can you picture how tiny that is? So, it really is about the quality, and not quantity, of colostrum. Your breasts will be producing teaspoons of colostrum rather than ounces in those first few days, so there really isn't anything to worry about.

Once your milk comes in, your baby's stomach capacity will also expand and be able to store around 1½ to 2 tablespoons of milk. This is one of the things that I think is so interesting, the expansion of your baby's stomach correlates with when your milk comes in, they happen around the same time as each other.

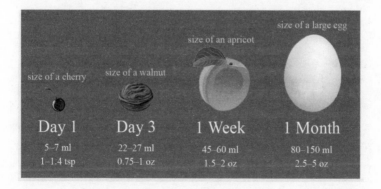

MY BREAST MILK IS JUST
RIGHT FOR MY BABY.

9

Breastfeeding Timeline

When I was breastfeeding Dakota, the first goal I set myself was getting to six months. I thought that's when she would want to start weaning onto solids and so I would stop then. That was what I thought was socially acceptable. I now often ask myself why I thought this.

My problem was, once I got to six months, I absolutely loved breastfeeding. I didn't want to stop and, most importantly, neither did my baby. *But wouldn't I be 'weird' if I carried on?* I thought to myself. None of my friends breastfed and anyone who did, had done it for a month or so. I felt like I was in unknown territory and was constantly being asked by people, 'When are you going to stop?' 'Oh, you aren't still breastfeeding, are you?' I would make jokes alongside them, but deep down, I had this huge desire to continue and so did my daughter, it seemed.

I started looking online to see what benefits there were for breastfeeding after six months and I learnt that there were so, so many! I used this information as my ammunition when people would ask why I was still breastfeeding past six months. Instead of saying defensively, 'Because me and my baby want to and it's none of your business', which is what I was thinking in my head, I would give them the facts behind breast-feeding, sharing my knowledge. I showed them I had another reason to do it (not just my pure love for it) because I felt judged.

My second time around with the twins, once I started breastfeeding, I was a lot more knowledgeable and 100 per cent comfortable and confident in my decisions. I could say proudly to anyone, 'I have no intention of stopping. Why would I? I'm happy and my girls are happy.' But it took my whole pregnancy, fuelled with insecurities from judgements made by small-minded people and lots of tears my end, to get to the stage of owning my choices and decisions and not caring about what others thought.

Once I started to share my breastfeeding journey on social media when the twins were a week old, the amount of positivity I received was amazing. So many mums all around the world told me that they respected my decisions, which filled me with love and confidence. Whether they breastfed or formula fed, they respected me and my choices, and that gave me the confidence to face people who were uneducated and unsupportive on the subject of breastfeeding.

I would love for every breastfeeding mum to feel as confident as I was when I was breastfeeding the second time around, but I know in reality that will not always be the case. With hormones, lack of sleep and often the hurdles to overcome with breastfeeding, you won't always feel fuelled with confidence to come back and stand up for yourself. As long as you are not influenced by what other people think or say, and feed how you want to feed your babies, that's the most important thing.

Here, I wanted to share with you a timeline of the benefits for breastfeeding, and not just for the first six months. If you are worried about comments from small-minded people, hopefully this will make you feel stronger and more confident in your decision.

First few days

Breastfeeding during the first few days helps your womb to start contracting back to its normal size (feels like period pains). During pregnancy and after you give birth, your body is producing colostrum – known as a mind-blowing superfood – for your newborn, which is designed to meet all your baby's exact needs for the first few days after birth. Below are some of the amazing things colostrum does:

- Coats your baby's stomach and intestines to keep germs out to prevent illness and possibly allergies
- Contains high concentrations of nutrients and antibodies, carbohydrates, protein and is low in fat (newborns can find fat difficult to digest)

- Mild laxative, helping your baby to pass their first stool (which is called meconium, and is made up of cells, protein, fats, mucus, amniotic fluid, bile and water.)
- Helps to reduce jaundice. Meconium stools are rich in bilirubin, a waste product of dead red blood cells, which is produced in large quantities at birth due to blood volume reduction
- Establishes beneficial bacteria in the digestive tract
- Kills harmful microorganisms and provides protection from inflammation

One month

- Helps to prevent digestive issues
- Lower risk of chest infections
- Hormones help you get back to sleep after night feeds
- At the six-week point, breastfeeding halves the risk of chest infections from now until around seven years old
- For premature babies, helps to prevent heart disease later in life

Two months

- The risk of getting Sudden Infant Death Syndrome (SIDS) is almost halved
- Reduced risk of food allergies by the age of three
- Helps prevent respiratory allergies

Three to four months

- Reduced risk of developing asthma

- Reduced risk of developing type 1 diabetes
- Mums still breastfeeding at this point may have a lower chance of postnatal depression (PND)

Six months

- Helps to prevent ear infections
- Reduces the chances of the mother getting breast and ovarian cancer
- There is 19 per cent less chance of childhood leukaemia
- Your baby is more likely to eat a range of different flavoured foods from tasting your milk
- Breast milk helps to digest new solid foods that are introduced into your child's diet
- Delays the return of the menstrual cycle
- Reduces the risk of you developing type 2 diabetes

Nine months

- You will have breastfed your baby through the fastest and most important brain and body development period
- Reduced risk of childhood obesity

Twelve months and beyond

- Your risk of ovarian and breast cancer reduces the longer you breastfeed
- Breastfed toddlers between the ages of one and three have been found to have fewer illnesses, illnesses of shorter duration and lower mortality rates

- Breastfeeding has shown the greatest gains for those children breastfed the longest
- Less likely to need orthodontic treatment and decreased risk of tooth decay
- The World Health Organization emphasises the importance of nursing up to two years of age or beyond:
  - Up to two years, more likely to have a high IQ
  - From 12 to 23 months, 448ml of breast milk provides:

    29 per cent of energy requirements

    43 per cent of protein requirements

    36 per cent of calcium requirements

    75 per cent of vitamin A requirements

    76 per cent of folate requirements

    94 per cent of vitamin B12 requirements

    60 per cent of vitamin C requirements[1]

The benefits of breastfeeding do not just finish at six, or even 12 months, and a lot of these advantages will last a lifetime. Breast milk changes continually through your breastfeeding journey to suit the needs of your baby, each and every step of the way. Not to mention saving your bank balance and time. If you want to do it, and can, then these are some excellent reasons to do so!

---

[1] Information from: https://www.nct.org.uk/sites/default/files/related_documents/reasons%20-to-be-proud_web.pdf

ANYONE OFFENDED BY
BREASTFEEDING IS
STARING TOO HARD!

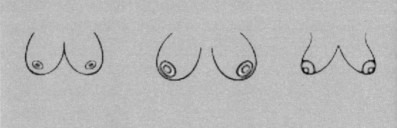

PART 3

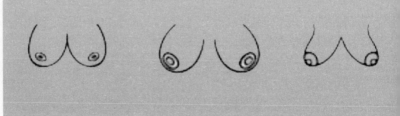

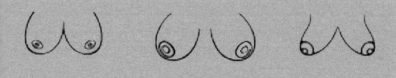

PROBLEMS, HURDLES & SOLUTIONS

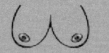 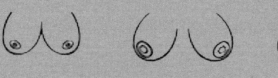

10

Hurdles to Overcome

Biting

When each of my girls started getting teeth, people would say, 'Ooh, are you going to stop now? You can't breastfeed when they have teeth, can you?' I must admit, when I had my eldest, this was something I was thinking in my mind at the time, purely because I didn't know any better. The problem was, I was not ready to stop breastfeeding and neither was my baby. So, I thought to myself, *I will just see how it goes and see just how horrendous it's going to be and if I can cope*. But that time just did not arrive. It didn't get horrendous once Dakota's teeth arrived – in fact, it felt the same as before she had any teeth at all!

Something that I now I know is if you are breastfeeding correctly, then you should not be able to feel your baby's teeth at all, even if they have a full set of gnashers. It's very important to know that it is PHYSICALLY IMPOSSIBLE TO BREASTFEED AND BITE AT THE SAME TIME. Your baby's tongue covers their bottom gums so once their teeth arrive (any time from birth to one year), their tongue will be covering their teeth. This means when they are feeding it would be impossible for them to bite, otherwise they would bite themselves.

While your baby is feeding, you are totally safe from being bitten. Now, you may read the above and think, *I'm sure I have heard of babies biting their mums*. Well, you would be correct: they can bite you, just not while they are actively breastfeeding. Here are some reasons why babies bite:

1. Normally, if babies are going to bite, it happens once they have finished feeding. You may not have even realised that your baby has finished feeding and this is when it can happen. They are slightly bored and no longer hungry (of course they can bite before they feed as well, it is just less common).
2. Maybe your baby is teething. Often, babies just want to clamp down on anything for a bit of a relief when teething. Unfortunately, sometimes that might be your nipple! The best thing is to have your little finger at the ready to pop in the corner of their mouth to unlatch the bite.
3. Maybe they are biting because they are wanting more attention. If you think this may be the reason, try looking your baby in the eye so they know they have your attention.
4. Your baby could have a cold or blocked nose and so might be having trouble breathing or swallowing. If you think this is the case, try sitting them up while you're feeding as this may make it easier.

Not every baby bites – some may only bite a few times and others may go through a biting stage. All three of my girls bit me a couple of times each. To stop this from happening, it's important to be consistent. Stop breastfeeding straight away, telling them a firm no, and also praise them when they are feeding and don't bite.

If your baby does bite you and clamps down (most babies won't do this), use your little finger in the side of their mouth to break the suction and help unlatch and say no firmly. If this doesn't work, then gently press your baby's face into your breast for a second, which will make it a little harder for them to breathe and they will automatically unclamp and open their mouth to breath[1].

Nursing strike

When babies start to refuse the breast, do not panic: this probably does not mean they are ready to wean and no longer want to breastfeed. It's easy to jump to conclusions and think this is the end of your breastfeeding journey but if your baby has been breastfeeding well and frequently and then suddenly refuses the breast, it is more than likely a breastfeeding strike.

Most nursing strikes are over as quickly as they started, around two to four days, but may go on for

---

[1] https://www.nct.org.uk/baby-toddler/feeding/common-concerns/breastfeeding-why-babies-may-bite-and-how-stop-it

longer. Nursing strikes normally happen for a reason like teething, or feeling under the weather – it could even be down to changing your perfume and they might not like the smell!

Whatever the reason, nursing strikes are difficult and emotional for you and your baby, no matter how laid-back and experienced you might be. It's important to try and encourage your baby to feed again and if they are not interested, try and turn it into some special skin-to-skin snuggles. Remember to make sure you pump every few hours or when they would normally feed – important as there is a risk of getting mastitis or blocked milk ducts (*see also* pages 111–13) – but obviously, it is also crucial to keep your milk supply up. If you do not have a pump, then you can definitely hand express, you should be shown in hospital how to do this. If you aren't then please ask and you can also watch great tutorials online, do check out: www.globalhealthmedia.org/portfolio-items/how-to-express-breastmilk/. The milk you express can be given to your baby in a beaker, cup or even a syringe, as well as a bottle, so they are still getting what they need.

Ways to encourage breastfeeding again:

1. Babies that are on a nursing strike when they are awake may feed when they are sleepy. Try as soon as they wake up from their nap/sleep, or when they are starting to fall asleep.
2. Have a bath with your baby and try breastfeeding in the bath, giving lots of skin-to-skin and attention.

Your breasts are there for when they want them and they may just latch on.

3. Be patient and try not to stress. Trying to force your baby to breastfeed will probably cause more harm than good. They want to feel relaxed and calm when breastfeeding, and so do you!

4. Try different positions, as maybe they are more comfortable in one position than another.

5. Babies can be distracted very easily, so try breastfeeding in a quiet, calm room, free from any distractions (maybe try in the dark also!).

6. Try co-sleeping, following safety guidelines, with no top on. Once again, like the bath, your breasts are readily available and with no pressure, they may just help themselves through the night! For lots of information and helpful videos do check out The Lullaby Trust website – they also offer great support for parents about safe sleep.

If it has been a few days, and none of the above is working, then please contact your local lactation consultant or health visitor, who can offer further advice more personal to you and your situation.

Blocked milk ducts & mastitis

The easiest example to use to describe blocked milk ducts is that your breasts might be making milk faster than your baby is effectively draining it. Maybe your child has started sleeping through the night, which means dropping feeds. Or, it might be caused by a poorly fitted bra or restrictive clothing, which means your milk can get backed up in your breasts. When this happens, the tissue around the ducts may become inflamed, swollen or tender.

Signs you have a blocked milk duct:

1. You might be able to feel a swollen lump, normally a bit like a marble, but it can also be more of a wedge shape
2. You may notice a red patch on your breast
3. Your breast may feel hot to touch and tender
4. Temperature under 38.5°C (101.3°F).

It's so important to keep feeding from your breast to avoid it getting infected and turning into mastitis. It can be really painful and it's so important to try and sort the situation as quickly as possible. Mastitis can happen when blocked milk ducts haven't cleared and become infected.

Signs you have mastitis are the same as blocked milk ducts but pain, heat and swelling is usually more intense, and you may now also be feeling some of the symptoms below which you wouldn't with blocked milk ducts:

1. Feeling generally unwell/flu-like symptoms
2. Temperature over 38.5°C (101.3°F)
3. Chills.

If you think you have blocked milk ducts, mastitis treatment is similar for both and the sooner you can resolve the blockage, the sooner you will feel better:

- Feed from your breasts as much as you can, making sure you alternate between breasts
- A cold compress will reduce inflammation
- Fill a sink with warm water, soak your affected breast and gently massage towards the nipple to help get your milk moving
- Lay in a warm bath, soak your breasts (and give yourself a break) and hand express (*see also* page 110)
- Put a flannel under warm/hot water, place it where the blockage is and massage to release milk (this worked wonders for me!)
- Change feeding positions with your baby's chin towards the blockage
- Rest as much as you can and stay hydrated
- Alternate paracetamol and ibuprofen every two hours (as long as you are safe to take it).

If any flu-like symptoms and your high temperature do not reduce within eight to 24 hours, call your doctor or dial 111 if it's out of hours. You may need antibiotics to help fight the infection.

Painful nipples

Breastfeeding will hopefully be enjoyable for you, so if your nipples are painful and crack and bleed, then this is a serious problem you need to look into. What would be great is to try and prevent your nipples from hurting in the first place.

The way your baby latches and their positioning are so important. If they have a poor latch, this can result in your nipples cracking – by far the most common reason for painful nipples. Remember, you and your baby are both learning and it can take some time to master breastfeeding, but practice and perseverance will get you there. Really look into how your baby is latched – are they in the correct position? Make sure your baby's lower lip is in a neutral position. It is so important that their latch is deep. It's crazy how far down your baby's mouth your nipple goes! As they are feeding, their latch might be slipping down and if that's the case, you can unlatch them and try again. Keeping your baby close and leaning back a bit will help prevent them slipping onto the nipple.

Maybe your baby has gotten used to a bottle or dummy and are finding it more difficult to latch well.

If your latch appears to be good and you are still experiencing pain or cracked nipples, make sure you find some breastfeeding support. It may be that your baby is tongue-tied. It is sometimes picked up in hospital, but it is often difficult to spot in the early days. An IBCLC or tongue-tie practitioner can do an oral and feeding assessment and will be able to suggest if a tongue-tie division would improve the situation.

Inverted & flat nipples

As long as your latch is correct and your baby is taking as much areola into their mouth as they can, then you really shouldn't have a problem. I had an inverted nipple, which I had pierced, then my body rejected the piercing so I had to take it out, resulting in that nipple becoming quite flat, but it was also a lot wider than my 'normal nipple'. This was the nipple that split with me as I had trouble latching Dakota, my eldest daughter, but once rectified, it was fine and we breastfed from it. I know a lot of mums with inverted nipples who have been able to feed successfully. Remember, you are breastfeeding, not nipple-feeding.

If you are struggling, then it's a good idea to maybe express for a few seconds before your baby latches on to draw the nipple out. You can also buy a little device called a nipple everter or you can make one from an old syringe. If your inverted nipple is quite severe then it's a good idea to practise deep-latch techniques. Also, look into getting a breast shield, which can be worn underneath your bra before you have your baby and in between feeds. They add a slight pressure to help draw the nipple out.

Thrush

Thrush is an overgrowth of the yeast organism *Candida albicans*. It is something that is always present in our bodies, but when we are ill, run down, tired, pregnant or taking antibiotics, it can overgrow and then cause thrush. It thrives in dark, moist areas, so leaking nipples going back into a bra and onto a moist breast pad can sometimes cause problems.

Signs you have thrush:

- Nipple pain (can be severe), burning, itching, sharp stabbing, pins and needles (breastfeeding should be pain-free after the initial attachment, thrush causes nipple pain after the feed)
- Inflammation of your nipple or areola
- Change in appearance of nipples: shiny, flaky, small blisters, white patches
- Irritation on your baby's mouth, white patches on their mouth or white coating on their tongue.

If you have thrush, you might want to stop breastfeeding, but even if your child isn't showing any symptoms, they may still have been exposed, so you will both need treatment. Book a doctor's appointment as soon as possible, so you can both get tested. You will both be given swabs to confirm thrush, and if it comes back positive you will likely be prescribed a gel for your baby's mouth and a cream for your nipple.

Although it is safe to breastfeed while you have thrush, it may cause pain in your baby's mouth and lips, so they might fuss more or avoid feeding. If you do miss feeds, continue to pump to keep your milk supply up, but you should not store expressed milk if you have thrush.

Tongue-tie

If you are experiencing pain when breastfeeding or maybe your baby isn't gaining weight, then hopefully, it will just be as simple as adjusting your position or latch. In some circumstances, it may be tongue-tie. Having a tongue-tie can stop your baby from being able to move their tongue freely, which means it can cause trouble and affect feeding. Normally, your midwife will tell you if they think your baby has tongue-tie, but sometimes it can be missed, so it's important if you are in pain or your baby is having poor weight gain to get this checked out by a lactation consultant (*see also* Support, 251).

Signs to look out for:

- Baby's tongue can't come out past their lips
- Heart shaped tongue, indentation at tip of the tongue
- Struggling to latch
- Unable to have a deep latch
- Makes a clicking sound when feeding
- Unable to stay latched on
- Poor weight gain
- Nipple flattened after feeding
- Painful feeds when latch is good
- Fussing at the breast.

Some babies have tongue-ties and will not need treatment. My eldest had a slight tongue-tie, which meant it took a while to get her to latch correctly but she gained weight OK. Once we corrected our latch and position, my nipples didn't hurt again after that. Others may need a tongue-tie division in order for the tongue to function effectively and for breastfeeding to work well. Make sure you see an IBCLC or tongue-tie practitioner who can do an oral and feeding assessment, and who can suggest whether further treatment may be appropriate.

Engorgement

When your milk 'comes in', your breasts can literally feel rock-solid, ready to overflow. Engorged breasts can feel painful, very sensitive and warm. With your milk coming in, it is common to have engorged breasts in the early days, and it normally only lasts around 24 hours. Because of the swelling, your nipples can flatten and areolas can stretch and feel hard, and this can make it more difficult for your baby to latch on. Some hand expression or massage can help soften the area. Some women may even experience a low-grade fever.

There are a few different reasons for engorgement, like feeding on a schedule, having a sleepy baby who may not be feeding frequently and expressing too much, or making more milk than you need. If you are cutting out feeds or stopping, sometimes if you do this too quickly without letting your breasts adjust this can cause engorgement.

There are plenty of things you can do to help:

- Feed often, eight to 12 times in 24 hours
- Hand express a little before you feed to soften your nipples (*see also* page 110)
- Listen for your baby's feeding cues, and feed on demand
- Allow baby to finish first breast before offering second breast
- Cold compress between feeds to help with swelling
- Warm compression when feeding to help milk flow (avoid adding warmth between feeds as it can add to the inflammation)
- Gentle massage towards your nipple before breast-feeding and whilst breastfeeding
- Find a good fitting bra, that's comfortable and can support you
- Drink to thirst and stay hydrated.

FUN FACT

Breast milk changes if your baby is ill

This is something that has always blown my mind! If you are breastfeeding and you are exposed to a virus, your breast milk will produce antibodies to help protect your baby from getting ill. If you are out and about and somebody sneezes on you, you then ingest their germs. Well, within 20 minutes, your milk will be producing antibodies to help your baby fight that particular virus. HOW AMAZING IS THAT? If your baby does get ill, research indicates that they pass on a cue through their saliva, which then in return sends a signal to your body to produce more milk with illness-specific antibodies[2].

Kissing your baby will also help their immune system. When you kiss your baby, you are 'sampling' the pathogens on their skin, which are then transferred to your lymphatic system, where you will produce antibodies to any bugs. These antibodies will then pass through your breast milk to your baby and boost their immune system.[3]

---

[2] https://www.ncbi.nlm.nih.gov/pmc/articles/PMC4334701/

[3] http://www.newbaby101.com.au/motherbaby-sharing-pathogens-goes-viral-on-facebook/

11

Re-lactation

Re-lactation is when you start breastfeeding again after a period of no breastfeeding, so this chapter is for you if you want to start over. You might have felt like you were ready to stop breastfeeding and then changed your mind, or maybe you were struggling and didn't think you were doing well but want to give it another go. Whatever the reason, you should know that it is possible. Plus, what have you got to lose by trying? Nothing. It's going to take some time, which will obviously differ from one breastfeeding mum to another, but it will be well worth it if this is something you want to do.

If your milk supply was in full swing once you stopped breastfeeding, it will probably take roughly the same amount of time that you have stopped breastfeeding for to start it up again. So, the longer you have stopped, the longer it will take to regain your milk. If your milk supply wasn't fully established or you stopped for a few months, then you may not be able to get a full milk supply back but you should still get good results.

In general, it is almost always possible to get some milk supply back and this is something important to remember if you are ever doubting your supply: women can re-lactate after months of not breastfeeding. Try not to worry when you first start trying to re-lactate about how much milk you can express – remember, any breast stimulation will be telling your body to produce more milk for the future, which is what you are after.

How to start

Check out the Facebook group 'UK Relactation and Adoptive Breastfeeding Support', where you can stock up on knowledge and information from mums who have done the same and expert voices, as well as mums lactating who are adopting their babies. How inspiring is that?! You will need to stimulate your breasts, which will send hormonal signals to your body to start up milk production. It may be easier if you only stopped breast-feeding a short time ago and you had a full milk supply in the past.

If your baby is willing to latch on, then put them to your breast every two to three hours. If they are looking for some comfort, put them on too – this will only add to helping build your milk supply back. Not all babies will be willing to latch after moving on to a bottle but do keep trying, it may take some time and persever-ance. You will need to give additional milk to begin with whilst your breasts begin to make more milk. Start hand expressing to begin with and then pumping once you begin to get some milk, preferably every two to three hours too (*see also* pages 63–64). If your baby is latching on, do this after every time they latch on and at least eight times in a 24-hour period. If you can, then at least once through the night as well, as this is when your levels of milk-making hormones are highest so will provide extra stimulation. If you can't manage the frequency then try as often as you can, but it will take longer to get your supply going again.

If your baby isn't latching on just yet, then hand express and pump every few hours. Also, looking into cluster pumping as a good option. Enjoy lots of skin-to-skin – this is so powerful in establishing breastfeeding and it can really help you with your re-lactation journey.

You may want to try some herbal supplements that help aid initiation and maintenance of breast milk. For more information do check out 'galactogogues' on The Breastfeeding Network website.

Keeping your baby fed while you are regaining your milk supply

While trying to build your milk supply back up, it's important that your baby is still fed, with either donor milk or formula. You could try paced bottle feeding, which can help your baby to re-latch onto your breast. It slows the pace of the milk flow, meaning your child will have to work harder for their milk – similar to if they were breastfeeding. You can gradually reduce the amount of substitute milk you give your baby as your milk supply increases. It is also a good idea to get some face-to-face advice from a lactation consultant.

FUN FACT

Breast milk changes at night

Your baby will get a different milk depending on the time of day. Breastfeeding in the morning will help to wake them up as at this time of day your breast milk contains natural stimulants. Whereas breastfeeding at night helps your baby to sleep, thanks to calming chemicals called nucleotides that reach their highest concentrations in your breast milk in the evening. Also, your night-time breast milk is rich in melatonin, which helps babies to develop their circadian rhythm and learn to differentiate night from day[1].

---

[1] www.llli.org/breast-milks-circadian-rhythms-2

MAYBE IT WON'T WORK
OUT, BUT MAYBE SEEING
IF IT DOES WILL BE THE
BEST ADVENTURE.

12

How Long Should I Breastfeed For?

When it comes to breastfeeding, there is no right or wrong length of time. The World Health Organization has put some guidelines in place based on their own scientific research[1], but I think it's very important to factor in your own wellbeing as it's a very personal decision and there are so many things to take into consideration.

In this chapter I'm going to give you as much information and support as I can to help you make the right decision for you and your baby, but please know this isn't a decision you have to make and stick to – things change all the time! I set myself a goal of six months with my first daughter, Dakota, and continued until 19 months, or you might set yourself a goal of a year and decide at six months that you would like to finish breastfeeding. This is your decision, you are in control and there are no right or wrong answers: you do what's best for you.

Personally, I think it's great to set yourself a goal as when you have a not-so-good day, it will hopefully

---

[1] https://www.who.int/mediacentre/news/statements/2011/breast-feeding_20110115/en/

remind you of where you would like to be and allow you to carry on to reach your target. But remember, your goal is not set in stone. I breastfed my twins for two years and four months and the thought of setting that goal when I was pregnant would have seemed so unrealistic and not a goal I would have wanted to stick to – it might even have put me off! But I just loved feeding my girls so much, we kept on going and going. I think most people who breastfed for an extended period didn't set out to do so and it was something that worked for them as they were enjoying it and so was their baby, so what was the point in looking to end?

As I always say, don't give up on a bad day because tomorrow could be your best. Of course, setting a goal might not work for everyone and it may add pressure that you don't need or want. If you are feeling more this way inclined, it's important to do what's best for you, always.

How to stop

So, you have chosen to draw your breastfeeding journey to a close, or you might need to because of different reasons. I know how emotional this can be – even if you are completely ready to stop, it can still be a sad time not only for you but also your baby. Make sure you are kind to yourself and slowly cut down feeds.

You could try mother-led weaning, which is where you slowly drop feeds. It's important if you drop one feed from your day that you wait for a few days for your body to adjust and your breasts to start producing less milk before you drop another. Remember, if you do this and your child is under 12 months then you need to replace that dropped feed with a bottle of formula, and if they are over 12 months with any whole animal milk (cow, goat, sheep) – make sure they are pasteurised. If your child has an allergy to animal milk protein then there are alternatives like, soya and oat. Please make sure you seek advice from a health visitor first if you want to use a milk alternative. You do not need to buy any special formula aimed at toddlers.

This is how I ended my first breastfeeding journey and we went straight on to beakers, as at 12 months most people start to wean off bottles so there is no need to buy them. Something else worth noting: if you are ending your journey with an older child, they do not need to substitute each feed with cow's milk as they are breastfeeding for so many more reasons than just to get milk and by this time they will be getting a lot of what they need from solids over a 24-hour period.

When we were doing mother-led weaning, the first feeds we dropped were the comfort feeds, the ones where they were fussing and just wanted to breastfeed not for food or drink but for comfort. I found these the hardest to stop, but once we had dropped them the next feeds became easier. The feed I planned to leave until last was their bed-time feed, but it just wasn't doable with our busy house and was too much of an inconvenience, so work out what works best for you and let it be a slow transition. I didn't experience any engorgement as every dropped feed I waited a good few days before we dropped the next.

There is another option, child-led weaning, where your baby/child decides when they are ready to stop breastfeeding. This is normally a very slow and gradual process, and is how my breastfeeding journey ended with the twins. I had already started mother-led weaning and slowly dropping my feeds down to once a day, which I was happy with. We still got to have that connection and bond and they were still getting a lot of goodness. Slowly, but surely, I started noticing they were missing that feed for a day or so and then eventually we were down to one feed a week. I could have continued happily this way, but before I knew it, a few weeks had passed. Our journey ended in December 2019 I wish I'd taken that last feed in, maybe had a photo taken. It makes me sad that I didn't know that was it, the end of our journey! I now substitute our breastfeeding connection with cuddles in bed every morning before we get up for the day and also reading on the sofa together. But I do miss the physical closeness and connection that breastfeeding brought to us.

It's important not to go cold turkey when breastfeeding as this can often produce mastitis and very engorged painful breasts (*see also* pages 111–13 and 118–19) as your milk supply has not had time to adjust. This can be incredibly painful and you could be quite unwell. Also, when you stop breastfeeding, your oxytocin – the love hormone – decreases, so you may feel sad and irritable or just generally quite low at a time that can already feel emotional. Even when I dropped my feeds very slowly, I really felt the affect and felt very sad and emotional about silly things. Be kind to yourself, take some time to acknowledge your feelings and think of new ways to get your oxytocin levels back up. Lots of cuddles, exercising and if you have time, new hobbies that are just for you.

FUN FACT

Breast milk changes flavour

What you eat and your diet can affect the taste of your breast milk. It has been suggested that breastfed babies are less fussy eaters once they start to eat solids because of their experience of flavours of foods you ate while breastfeeding[2].

---

[2] https://www.llli.org/breastfeeding-info/foods/

13

Breastfeeding Twins, Triplets & More

Obviously, this chapter might not apply to you, so feel free to skip! I have experience of breastfeeding twins and it's a really interesting topic, so do stick around if you are intrigued and want to know more.

If you are pregnant with twins and are reading this wondering whether it is actually possible to breastfeed, let me tell you, no, let me SHOUT through these pages, 'YES, YES, YOU CAN DO IT!!' It makes me feel emotional writing that. When I found out I was pregnant with twins, the first thing I said, after a few choice swear words (and then, of course, celebrating my pregnancy), was, 'That means I won't be able to breastfeed.' After building such a love and passion for breastfeeding with my eldest, the thought of not being able to breastfeed my new babies really hit me.

After going and telling all of my family face to face that I was having twins and already being told by certain family members, 'Don't even think about breastfeeding twins' and 'Don't be silly, that's just not going to be possible' (all from women who had never breastfed themselves, I might add), I drove home with even more self-doubt and worries. I remember from that moment feeling like I was going to be seen as a freak every time I told someone I was going to breastfeed twins. I even tried to play it down because I didn't want to be met with negativity, or to be mocked, so I would lie and say, 'I might try it, we'll see.' If I could go back now, I would stand there so proudly and say, 'YES, I'm going to try and breastfeed my girls exclusively! I've done it once and my body will do it again.'

After I got home from telling my family the news of having twins, I researched, researched and researched some more. I started off thinking maybe I could combi-feed as that way, I still got my dream to be able to breastfeed again even if it wasn't exactly as I would have wanted it. The more I found out and researched (and I also joined the Facebook group Breastfeeding Twins and Triplets UK), I knew that this was actually possible: I could certainly try to breastfeed my twins exclusively and I was going to give it my all to have the best crack at it. Silently but confidently, I knew I could do it. I didn't buy any bottles or formula as backup, I had made my decision and I was going to breastfeed and that was that! On the Breastfeeding Twins and Triplets UK Facebook group there are mums with triplets who were still breastfeeding exclusively past one year and if they could do it, so could I! Why not? I had two boobs, two arms, two babies . . . Our bodies had made two babies at the same time, so it would be possible to produce enough milk to feed them as well.

Congratulations, you are one of the lucky chosen ones, is how I felt. But I was also crapping myself and I had a lot of self-doubt, thinking about how tough it was going to be. If I could go back and talk to myself then, I would want to change my whole way of thinking. As I can't go back in time, I'm going to tell YOU instead. You can do this, yes, it's tough and some of the early days were really tough, but now I also know twin mums who find the whole thing a breeze (I was not one of those!). I remember when I was pregnant, thinking how many times I would be breastfeeding through the night, but when it comes to it, you just go through the motions, you adapt and get on with it.

I wish I hadn't spent my pregnancy worrying about the what ifs, as it doesn't change the outcome, but it does make you stressed when you don't need to be. You need to surround yourself with people who are all for you breastfeeding multiples and if those closest to you don't agree, tell them they don't have a choice in the matter! You will probably have people say to you, 'But if you formula feed, I can help.' But the person doing most of the feeding is you! Once they go home and they pop in once a week, who's left doing the work? You are! It goes without saying that if you want to formula feed, then of course that's absolutely fine and the best thing for you. Remember it is no one else's choice how you feed your babies, the thought of having twins is already stressful enough, let alone feeding them in a way that someone else is encouraging you to if that isn't what you want.

What I'm trying to say is, just because you may have found out you are having twins or triplets, don't think this means you can't breastfeed because you absolutely can. There's a higher chance your babies will be born early or premature, there is also a greater chance of birth interventions as well, but your body is made to adapt and it will work out. With some perseverance from yourself, stocked up on knowledge and the support from the people around you, or even from an online community, you can do this!

Remember, if you read Chapter 3: Understanding Milk Production (pages 53–65), you will know it is all about supply and demand. When you have twins, you also have more placental tissue than if you were having a single baby, and then once again, even more placental tissue when you have triplets. The good thing about that is the more placental tissue you have, the more milk-making tissue your body creates. Proof once again from our bodies that you can do this!

First steps when you are pregnant with multiples

1. Make it known to your midwife and everyone around you that you want to breastfeed. Every health professional I met, from the sonographer, the team that helped me deliver the twins, the consultant, the

paediatrician who saw me the day after (knowing me, I probably told the cleaner on the ward) – everyone knew that was what I wanted to do. Hopefully, if you tell the midwife looking after you when you are pregnant, they can give you support and information beforehand.

2. Look into colostrum harvesting. Speak to your midwife about this – it should be offered at all hospitals and be discussed with you between 26 and 30 weeks – but if it is not mentioned, make sure you ask about it. As I said earlier, colostrum is the first milk that your body produces. It is full of goodness and contains antibodies that help fight against infection while a baby's immune system is developing. Very important for any baby, but especially babies from a multiple birth as they are more than likely to be premature.

You should be given 1ml syringes to collect your colostrum from the hospital but you can also buy them online for around £10 for 100. You can start hand expressing from 36 weeks, or around a week before a planned delivery. This would have helped me so much after the girls' birth. If your babies' blood sugars are low (common in multiple births), it takes the pressure off after giving birth as you have a little help in hand. If your babies do come early and you have not had time to harvest colostrum, do not panic: you will be able to start hand expressing immediately after birth. If not, you can ask your hospital for donor breast milk. Some hospitals do not supply this – mine didn't, so they did formula top-ups. Just make sure to always offer the breast first, and set up a plan to help get back to the goal of breastfeeding

3. Buy a breastfeeding pillow. I bought a normal breastfeeding pillow and there are many which are made specifically with twin mums in mind. They are all different depths, so it's good to do some research to figure out what is best for you. This website, www.breastfeedingtwinsandtriplets.co.uk, has some great information on each pillow to help you decide what will hopefully work best for you and your babies (*see also* Helpful Products, page 166). Breastfeeding pillows help to prevent slouching, which really helps to avoid a bad back. They can be quite pricey but you can always look on second-hand selling pages online, as well as breastfeeding twin and triplet pages and other bidding sites online (most have washable covers).

4. Find out about local breastfeeding groups and lactation consultants. You have two mouths to feed around the clock in the early days, so it's very important that any problems that may arise get sorted quickly. Something I recommend to mums that come to me is to speak with the amazing Kathryn Stagg, who is a lactation consultant and twin specialist. She does Skype or phone calls and you will not be able to find someone better to speak to at the drop of a hat. (*See also* Support, page 251.)

5. Join the amazing Facebook group, 'Breastfeeding Twins and Triplets UK'. Even if you do not have a Facebook account, I highly recommend you sign up, just to be able to join this group. This has been one of the most important factors of my breastfeeding journey with the twins. You will be truly inspired by watching everyone's breastfeeding journeys as well as learning SO much from other people's posts, sharing in their problems and seeing their real-life experiences.

6. Be positive. Once you make the decision to breast-feed twins, do not let doubt creep in. Own your decision and be confident that you know your body can breastfeed twins/triplets/more. Positivity is one of the key things to make this journey successful. Make sure you do all the research you can to stock up on information to solidify your decision and con-fidence in your choice.

7. Be flexible in how you feed your babies. When I was pregnant with twins, I thought I was always going to tandem feed (*see* pages 90–93) as it made sense that it would be easier and quicker than not. Then when my girls arrived, I ended up finding that feed-ing them separately was something I enjoyed more as I got the one-on-one bonding and they were both very quick feeders. I tended to tandem feed more in the day when I was more awake and could get into position more easily. Be prepared how you think might be easier or better for you might not

actually be the case, so it's good to try different ways to find out what works for you.

8. Play it by ear when it comes to who has what boob! Another decision I made when I was pregnant was to designate a twin to a boob. After a while, I noticed one of my breasts was getting a lot larger than the other, so then I swapped boobs and thought I would try a weekly shift. But then the opposite boob got bigger, so I realised one of my twins was a much more effective feeder than the other (she was a lot smaller and had some catching up to do). I decided to alternate breasts every 24 hours and some mums alternate every feed. There is no right or wrong way, just trial and error and figuring out what works best for you.

9. Do not underestimate how hard the early days can be. It is tough, it is relentless, it can be non-stop, but after six weeks, after that big growth spurt, I find that point is such a breakthrough and you will be thankful you stuck it through. If you put in the groundwork and try to get through the tough part in the early days, it becomes so much easier and it pays off.

I gave myself six weeks of basically being house-bound. During this time, I started a new boxset, got through lots of chocolate and we breastfed a lot. Sometimes for hours. Again, at 12 weeks, everything got a lot easier – I started noticing patterns in the twins' sleeping habits so I felt like I was getting a little bit of control over my days. But sometimes in the early days, it was horrendous. I don't want to scare you, but I think it's also very important to prepare you so you go into this knowing there is a good chance you aren't going to be a natural and it will take a lot of determination and perseverance.

10. Then again, don't underestimate how amazing and easy it becomes after the hard part! I would never be able to put into words how amazing my breastfeeding journeys were with all of my girls. Every tear, cracked nipples, cluster feed, engorged breast, for me it was all worth it, because the amazing part of breastfeeding overrides that tenfold. Plus, it becomes so easy, not having to remember bottles as you're running out of the house, or going to bed and forgetting you haven't sterilised enough bottles. Once you've got to grips with breastfeeding, your breasts are there and ready to go.

11. Take plenty of pictures and videos! I have a lot of photos of me breastfeeding the girls, mainly tandem feeding, and I only have one video of me breastfeeding in a supermarket(!), and I regret not getting more. This will be one of the most incredible journeys of your life, so make sure you document it.

FUN FACT

Breast milk adapts to baby's temperature
Your breasts can tell your baby's temperature!
Really, it's true. In return, your breast milk will
adjust by either warming or cooling, depending
on your child's needs. Your breast can even
detect a one-degree variation in your baby's
temperature[1].

---

[1] https://www.charlotteobserver.com/living/health-family/moms/article93194807.html

14

Breastfeeding in Public

The thought of breastfeeding in public can feel a bit daunting and scary, especially if you have never done it before. With my eldest in the early days, I used to feel anxious about latching her on, making sure my milk didn't squirt everywhere or she didn't decide to unlatch and start looking around. I was always covered up with a muslin cloth. But after a while, it just became second nature and I didn't think twice about feeding anywhere, anytime.

When I found out I was pregnant with twins, I remember crying my eyes out to my husband (clearly hormonal), saying, 'How am I going to breastfeed twins in public? I want to breastfeed them so much, but the thought of tandem feeding in public, I just won't leave the house!' Lewis then said something to me that was so simple, and so obvious, but it had just never crossed my mind, 'Feed them individually, one at a time, and it will be like breastfeeding a singleton.' Just like that, I stopped crying and I couldn't believe I hadn't thought of it myself, something so simple that made so much sense, I felt my worries melt away right there and then.

I did end up tandem feeding in public, but it wasn't until the girls were 18 months. When we did it, did we get some funny looks? I don't know, I wasn't looking at them. And if anyone had a problem with me breastfeeding in public, well then obviously they were looking too hard at me feeding my children! Something that I have always wondered when people don't like mums breastfeeding in public: they have two choices, listening to a baby screaming (and you can hardly shut that noise out of your ears), or carrying on with your normal activities and not staring. I know which I would rather.

I have breastfed in the queues at Disney World, on the beach, in restaurants, shops, aeroplanes, trains . . . If the girls needed feeding, I breastfed, anywhere, anytime. It is a great way to keep a baby calm when travelling – especially if you are flying. I would tandem feed the girls at take-off and landing, and then throughout the flight when they needed it. (I always felt like breastfeeding was my secret weapon to successful flights with all three of my girls.)

Some tips on feeding in public

I didn't buy any breastfeeding clothes, I just wore vest tops underneath everything. I would pull my top up and my vest down. In the summer, all of my dresses were wrap dresses or they buttoned up. If you would feel better and more confident being covered then you can buy special breastfeeding cover-ups, or use a swaddle or muslin cloth.

It's so easy to overthink things and worry about them, but when it comes to it, it doesn't really need to be that complicated. Remember, practice makes perfect. It may be daunting at the start, but that feeling won't last long. You'll look back and won't believe how much you overthought the situation and you'll be so proud of how far you've come.

Know your rights

Just to give you a little bit of backup, and hopefully help you to feel more confident breastfeeding in public, there are laws in the UK that protect women breastfeeding in public. Mums do not have to cover up while breastfeeding and it's a criminal act to stop a mother breastfeeding in public.

THERE IS NOTHING
BETTER THAN TIME
SPENT NOURISHING
MY BABY.

15

Partner Bonding

So many women who want to breastfeed worry about their partner not feeling included or missing out on feeding their baby. Personally, this wasn't something I was concerned about (sorry, Lew!), it just didn't cross my mind. I remember in making the decision that I wanted to breastfeed I did ask my husband how he felt not being able to feed his babies and he was totally fine with it, and 100 per cent supported me in breastfeeding our daughters. After all, there are so many other ways for partners to bond with their baby and feel included.

I had people say to me, 'But you won't have any help through the night.' My husband has a manual job Monday to Friday, so five nights a week, I wouldn't have been able to wake him to help me anyway. For me, it seemed pointless having him help when it would only be for two nights a week and it was so easy for me to put them on my boob and put them back in bed again without either of us having to get up to make bottles. To make sure we split the task equally of looking after our babies, however, I used to say to Lew, 'You do bum and I'll do boob.' For the first two weeks while he was off work on paternity leave, and at weekends, if they pooed in the night, that was his job! And let me tell you, between two newborn babies, there could be a lot of poos . . .

Ways for partners to bond with baby

You have been through something massive together, creating a new family unit. Enjoy these moments and get involved as much as you can:

- Just because your partner is breastfeeding, there's no reason why you also shouldn't have skin-to-skin contact with your baby. Skin-to-skin has so many amazing benefits – it calms them and you, helps babies to cry less, stabilises their heart rate. Lay on the sofa, take your top off and place your baby on your chest for lots of cuddles. They will feel calm and safe listening to your heartbeat.
- Bath your baby for more skin-to-skin and a lovely bonding experience. As they get older, bath-time becomes really fun for them and also for you in return. Once your baby has been bathed, you could do some baby massage after you have dried them with baby moisturiser and they will soon get to know your touch.
- Baby wearing: you could wear a sling and go for a walk with your baby. They will feel safe, protected and close to you. It's a great way of bonding, especially as it is hands-free.

- Sing: your baby will love to hear the sound of your voice and will soon recognise who you are by what you sound like. The sooner they hear your voice, the sooner your bonding begins, so feel free to start when they are in the womb!

- Play: whether it's peekaboo, tickles or a baby rattle. Parents play differently with their babies, so this is a great opportunity for you to bond with them in a specific way.

- Read: have them on your lap, snuggled in a comfy chair, or in bed. This has more benefits than just bonding, it helps them to start getting an attention span as well as remembering things. Your baby won't have a clue what you are reading, but once again, they will feel comforted by your voice.

- Put your baby to bed: if you've been at work all day and haven't spent time with your baby, this will be a lovely way for the two of you to have some one-on-one time together.

- Separating out tasks: my husband and I did bum and boob! Delegate jobs.

- Winding: you can wind your baby after a feed. Not all breastfed babies need to be winded, but I found all three of mind did. This is a great way for you to still be part of the breastfeeding process.

- Cuddle: have a big family cuddle while your partner is breastfeeding. It's peaceful and relaxing for you to be all together and your baby will know that you are there as part of that. What better way to bond than the whole family doing it together?

Alex Galbally, partner to Charlotte (read about Charlotte's story in chapter 26, 'Real Mums, Real Stories')

I guess the classic dad feeling when your partner is breastfeeding is to feel like a bit of a spare part! I think I felt like this with my son Henry at times, although being mine and Charlotte's first child, I didn't really know what was going on. Also, I don't think I realised how important it is to a woman to breastfeed. I tried my best, offering cups of tea, grabbing the breastfeeding pillow, foot rubs, but I think the most important role as a dad when baby is being breastfed is to support the mum, mentally more than anything.

I didn't learn this first time round mainly because Charlotte cracked on with it without much fuss, apart from the odd grumble about sore nipples or lack of sleep. It wasn't until we had the girls and mainly due to the medication she was on, as well as the dynamics of trying to breastfeed three children at once when you only have two boobs, that I saw how much it meant to her to breastfeed.

When I saw the pressure she was under and how much easier it would be for her to just stop and bottle feed the girls, meaning I could do it as well, I just tried to encourage her to stop. She was so upset and felt such a failure, it was at that moment that it resonated with me just how important it is for some women (on that note, I think mothers have the right to do whatever they think is right for them and their child when it comes to breastfeeding).

When Charlotte finally gave in and stopped breast-feeding, it took her a while to come to terms with it. That was the moment I knew I needed to step up and surround her with positive support. Having three babies meant we both had to nail some sort of routine and structure which, thank goodness, we did.

When little Jimmy came along in September 2019, Charlotte was always going to breastfeed him in the same way she did Henry. But I felt different this time: I knew what it meant to her, I also knew that while tea and support are important, I wanted to be more hands-on and involved. I burp Jimmy once Charlotte has fed him, I then change his nappy while she has a rest, etc. This way, we feel more like a team. We also obviously have four other children, so sometimes I will occupy them so Jimmy can have his feed in peace.

As a man and a dad, I think it's easy to feel pushed to the side and there is a temptation to be relaxed about everything and let the mum worry about it. I found that not letting this be the case has given me such a better bond with my children, also a better relationship with them. I am a big, hairy, heavily tattooed man who loves football and beer – but not as much as I love being there for my wife and children when they need me.

16

How Can My Family Help?

I'm writing this to your mum, your friend, your nan . . . whoever it may be that might not have breastfed and would like to know how they can help. There's nothing more empowering to a new mum who wants to breast-feed than those closest to her supporting her decision, encouraging her and allowing her to make her own choices. **I cannot emphasise this enough.** I know how exciting it is when someone close to you has a baby and you will probably want to be involved and help out as much as you can.

So many mums feel guilty and angry when they stop breastfeeding before they are ready. One of the big-gest reasons why is due to lack of support from those closest to them. It's not always a deliberate thing, but can be down to someone's lack of knowledge. Mums who breastfeed for longer are normally those who feel confident and empowered by the people around them. This was certainly the case for me and something I will be eternally grateful for with my partner, friends and family. I will also, unfortunately, never forget those close to me who actively tried to discourage me and argued against my decision to breastfeed, they added a lot of stress and upset when they had no need to.

I knew on my breastfeeding journey the people I would go to and count on when I was struggling who would lift me up with just a few words of encouragement and then there were people I would not want to speak to as their only solution was formula. If someone I cared for was breastfeeding, I know what person I would want to be for them – the one they called upon and felt safe speaking to with their struggles and not the opposite. This also works the same way for someone I cared for who is formula feeding and having a tough day with it. I would always want them to know they could come to me with no judgement or discouragement and they will only be met with empathy and encouragement. So, be comfortable around her breastfeeding: this will help her to feel relaxed and if she's relaxed, then her baby will sense it too; be their voice of support. If a problem arises, and they still want to breastfeed, help them find a solution: call the National Breastfeeding Helpline (0300 100 0212) or find a local lactation consultant. You can also do your own research on recommended online sites just to show your support even more, and how you value and respect their decision to breastfeed.

Babies need a lot of care and dedication, but so too do new mums. If you look after her, this will only help her to look after her baby too. It has a domino effect. Make sure she is eating and drinking, as she will be so preoccupied making sure her baby's needs are met, through sheer exhaustion, she will often forget about her own needs. So, that can be your job. Offer to look after her baby while she naps and promise you will wake her up when they want feeding. Help with housework – let's face it, if anything's going to take a backseat, it's that! Cook some meals too for storing in the fridge and freezer.

Some babies just do not want to be put down between feeds, so you could be the person in between giving lots of cuddles, having bonding time, changing nappies, offering to bath the baby, etc. Let Mum have some time to bathe, too! I think all new mums struggle to find the time to look after themselves and this is a great way of being able to do that.

It's so important that the new mum in your life trusts you and knows you respect her decision with regards to how she has decided to feed her baby. I know I wouldn't want to leave my child with someone that was discouraging of me breastfeeding and who didn't support my decision. Read earlier on in this book for advice and knowledge about hunger, cluster feeding, how quickly babies feed. Understanding breast milk intake is more complex than looking at the ounce mark on a bottle! You will also find earlier on in this book reasons why babies want milk – including hunger, thirst, to feel safe or for comfort, or simply to sleep. There are many more reasons than baby just being hungry. That's why it's important to not just suggest formula when you think maybe breast milk isn't enough. If her baby is gaining weight and having wet nappies, then this is a really good indication that the new mum's breast milk is doing an amazing job.

Breastfeeding can be considered a food, a medicine and a signal all at the same time. Something great for you to do is educate yourself so read books (already nailing that one!), research online, then when your partner/friend/family member does have struggles, you will be able to help them through those tough times. If you are educated in breastfeeding, you may be the best support she can ask for.

Last, but not least, tell her how proud you are of her! There will be days in every new mum's journey that may be really difficult and she might be feeling overwhelmed. Just a few kind, encouraging words from the people closest to her has more impact than you may realise!

17

I Want Some Freedom Back!

Breastfeeding your baby might end up being one of the best journeys of your life, but that doesn't take away from the fact that it's a huge commitment and one not to be underestimated or played down. Just like motherhood.

Breastfeeding is a full-time job, but so too of course is formula feeding. For me personally, the thought of bottle feeding was more of a hardship than breastfeeding: remembering to buy formula in the midst of my forever growing baby brain (it's a real thing, I felt like I had double baby brain after the twins) and then the sterilising and preparing for everything to be ready for each feed. I always thought that with breastfeeding, it doesn't matter how disorganised or forgetful you are, your breasts are attached to you and milk is readily available at the perfect temperature.

But what if you want a breather? What about when you fancy a night out with some friends, to do anything other than have to clean poo-ey nappies, or you'd like to rekindle some romance with your partner and have a date night? What then? Your breasts are attached to you, so you can hardly hand them over to someone else to take over!

The second time around, I knew what I was committing to when I decided I wanted to breastfeed my twins. I knew it was going to be very short-lived, having to feed around the clock with a baby attached to me, because before you know it, that stage is over and you do get some more freedom back. I remember feeling quite protective over my girls and that even though I may have wanted a break and craved some normality, I didn't actually want to leave the house without them. Of course, it is also normal to feel fine about leaving them to get some time for yourself, which is so important.

From about 12 weeks, you will start to notice a pattern in your baby's sleeping behaviour. At this stage for me with the twins, we started having set nap times and I knew how long they would sleep for. The girls may have only slept for two hours at a time, but that was all I felt I needed to nip out for some lunch with a friend, maybe a bit of retail therapy round the shops, or a nice dinner with my husband, while my mum had the girls. From six months, it became easier still as they started solids and had a beaker with water, so then it got even easier to have that break. Twelve weeks and six months might seem like a long time to wait for a break, but blink and before you know it, you're there. Just because this worked for me and that's how I felt doesn't mean you should feel the same though. You are entitled to want a break and some 'me time' whenever you feel the time is right; there really is no wrong or right here.

In the first few weeks, it's essential to feed on demand to help establish your supply, so if there's a reason you do need to be away from your baby in those early weeks then make sure you pump every two hours to avoid hindering your supply. Any pump will be fine for the occasional bottle and even hand expressing will work. If you are going to be pumping more long term, or going back to work early, then a hospital grade pump would be best. You can rent these or buy one on Amazon – both options should come with the option of next day delivery!

How can I get my breastfed baby to take a bottle?

Some babies will take a bottle absolutely fine first time and are able to switch between breast and bottle. Others might seem to prefer to breastfeed and even absolutely refuse to feed from a bottle. This obviously makes life difficult when you have plans to go out, or are thinking about going back to work. Here are some ways to try and encourage your breastfed baby to take a bottle:

- Stay calm: the first time I tried the twins with a bottle, I was planning on being away from them at around seven months as I was a bridesmaid at my friend's wedding. I thought it was important to try them with a bottle of my expressed breast milk before we went. I envisioned the moment of trying something new with the girls and was quite looking forward to this new experience with them, it did not go as I thought it would. They were both extremely unhappy to even try, so it was quite stressful on my part and theirs. Accept that they might not take the bottle first time and it could take some time and perseverance. Remember, your baby will get the vibe from you if you are stressed and agitated, so stop and try again.

- Get someone else to try: babies can smell your milk and if they can see you, they might get frustrated at not having what they are used to.
- Try different bottle teats: some teats are made to be similar to mothers' breasts, which can help your baby to still latch as they would when breastfeeding. There are teats of different firmness, widths, lengths, fast or slow flows – it's a bit of a minefield to be honest, but it's all based on trial and error.
- Try different positions: they may like to feed in the same positions you would put them in to breastfeed, or they might prefer to try a brand-new position as a bottle is also new to them.
- Experiment with different temperatures of milk: they may like it warm to replicate the breast or prefer it cold – try both.
- Don't wait until your baby is hungry and frustrated, but it's just as important not to try when they are not hungry, so go for somewhere in the middle! I know this totally sounds like a minefield, but just practise looking out for these instances.

- Maybe you could give a teat a go when your baby is asleep, safely.
- Movement: give them a little jiggle when you are trying them with a bottle.
- Try using a cup instead. This can be more successful with an older baby (past four months). An open cup or free-flowing sippy cup often works well.

18

Going Back to Work

If you're going back to work and would like to continue to breastfeed then please know that this is absolutely possible. You should not have to end your journey because of work. How old your baby is going to be when you go back to work will determine whether you may want/need to express while at work. Hopefully, your place of work will have a plan set up for breastfeeding mums and if they don't, then have a chat with them to help them put one in place.

Over six months

Once your baby is six months and having good food and water intake, you really do not have to do much to prepare. You can pump at work and if you're not too uncomfortable, your breasts will adjust to your new schedule and your baby will get everything they need from your breast milk during your new working hours. Once you're home from work, more than likely your baby will want to breastfeed straight away and it's a really lovely way for you two to connect, and what a lovely welcome home from your day at work. This is called reverse cycling, when your baby feeds more at night than during the day. They will make up for the milk they missed in the day and will consume more milk at night, and they will either want to breastfeed more or for longer feeds than usual.

Once your baby is on solids and having sufficient meals and water, then this is when you do not need to worry about pumping. Your child can feed and get everything they need around your working hours. Your breasts may feel a little uncomfortable though and you may want to express to feel more comfortable. Do not be surprised when you walk in through the door and your baby wants to feed a lot. (They will likely be craving that connection with you as they have missed you through the day and you will probably feel the same way.)

You may decide you would like to pump at work so you can give your baby a bottle/cup of expressed milk whilst you are away.

Under six months

This will take more planning as your baby won't be on solids or having water yet, so will still be needing milk regularly. If you cannot visit your child during your workday or they cannot be brought in to you, then you can express milk or combi-feed (formula when you are at work, breastfeed at home). You will choose what is right for you and your family, and remember not to let anyone influence you in this decision.

At work, there should be somewhere you can feel comfortable expressing (some people do it at their desk). Ask about this before you return to work, as some work places will never have had to accommodate a mother who is still breastfeeding. Whatever you feel comfortable with is important and will also help your milk to flow. How much you express and how many times a day is totally personal to you and dependent on how many feeds your baby will be missing. Also, like when you feed your baby, you shouldn't have set times, so when you express at work, this too doesn't have to be at exact times. It's good to check with your employer where you can store your milk in a fridge.

Just like breastfeeding, expressing is a skill. If you are having any worries or troubles, or looking for advice, then I recommend speaking to the La Leche League, Association of Breastfeeding Mothers, Breastfeeding Network, Lactation Consultants of GB, NCT, or National Breastfeeding helplines (*see also* Support, pages 249–53). They are some breastfeeding organisations that are able to give face-to-face support to breastfeeding mums, or over the phone or on the internet. Your breast milk will fluctuate and by the end of your working week, your milk supply may drop a little bit. Some skin-to-skin and continuing feeding when you can will make your milk flow a lot freer. Remember, your milk is like a tap and is made on a supply-and-demand basis. Please read the chapter on Understanding Milk Production in Part 2 of this book (pages 53–65). If you are finding your milk supply is starting to diminish, speak to your employer about potentially changing some working conditions so you are able to help build up your supply again. On days where you are at home, your baby is likely to still want to feed as normal and feed from you through the day.

Maximise breastfeeding directly and make sure child care doesn't give a bottle just before you are going to pick up baby, breastfeed all feeds when you are together, let baby cluster feed if they wish, allow lots of night feeds (reverse cycling).

The law for breastfeeding mums at work

Returning to work doesn't mean you have to stop breastfeeding and it's your decision when you would like to stop. Before you go back to work, I suggest giving your employer a written letter in which you state that you are still breastfeeding and want to continue to do so upon returning to work. They will hopefully conduct a specific risk assessment for you to do so. It is up to the discretion of your workplace if they provide suitable facilities where pregnant and breastfeeding mothers can rest. Please check with your direct line manager or HR department who needs to see this written letter and where it is going.

The Health and Safety Executive (HSE) recommends that it's good practice for employers to provide a private, healthy and safe environment for breastfeeding mothers to express and store milk. The women's toilets are not a suitable place to express breast milk![1]

---

[1] https://www.nhs.uk/conditions/pregnancy-and-baby/breastfeeding-back-to-work/

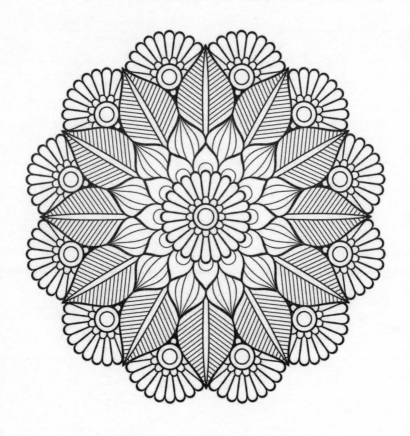

Colour in these Mandala drawings to help you relax, unwind and feel a deeper connection with yourself.

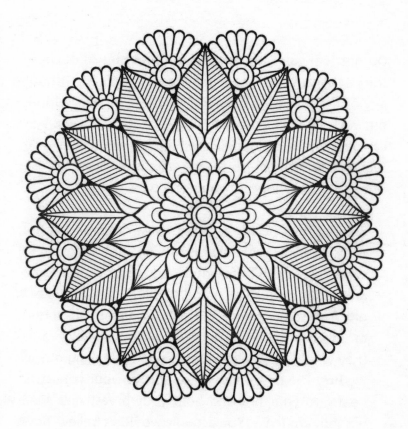

19

Helpful Products

Do not feel you have to rush out and buy all of these things, because of course you can breastfeed without any of the following products. These items are helpful, but with services often offering next-day delivery, you can get helpful things delivered really quickly when you feel you need them, so there really is no need to rush out and spend money if you don't have it now.

1. Breast pads: I personally think these are great! In the early days, all I remember is leaking a lot. It's good to experiment with different brands, as of course some are better than others, and to find what you like. I did find some where the edges were really rough on my skin or they didn't stick well with my bra so they would move and I would end up leaking out of my bra. The best ones will be soft on your skin, stick neatly to your bra and hold your breast milk well without any leaks. You actually wouldn't believe how much milk they can hold! But remember, it's good to keep your nipples dry as it will help keep bacteria at bay, which will help to prevent sore nipples, thrush or mastitis, so make sure you change pads regularly.

2. Nipple cream: Great for cracked and sore nipples! It's good to start using nipple cream before your nipples actually crack (if they crack at all). I know people who swear by Vaseline, which is a cheaper alternative. Also, if your nipples do crack, expressing some of your breast milk onto them is known to help as your milk has healing properties, plus it's free. Woohoo, winner!

3. Breast pumps: You might not plan on expressing, so this is something I would suggest to wait and see if you actually need one. For me, when one of my nipples cracked on my first breastfeeding journey, I found it less painful to pump than to breastfeed, so I was able to pump to keep up my breast milk supply without it hurting my nipples as much. I just used a very cheap ordinary manual pump which I found to be very effective and I would also hand express (*see also* page 110) if I found pumping too painful, which of course doesn't cost a thing.

When I had the twins, I really wanted to up my milk supply as their weight was so low. I would breastfeed them both and then after, I would express each breast so I kind of tricked my body into needing more milk. I did end up upgrading to an electric pump from a hand pump, which I loved, I found this so much easier to pump if I was out of the house and needed to express. Also, if you are in hospital and need a pump, they will be able to loan you one for the time you are there.

Hospital pumps are more powerful and more effective than a personal pump. They mimic your baby's natural stimulation, they are also a closed system, which means they have a barrier so they cannot get contaminated and can be used by more than one person. (If you are in hospital you will be given your own attachments.) They are stronger and are great if you are pumping to help increase your milk supply.

4. Breast milk bags/storage: If you do pump, it's good to keep your expressed breast milk and put it in a bag in the freezer. One of the shelves in my freezer is full of pumped breast milk. They have only been used a few times – like when I had a night away, I had a stash ready and waiting (and then I would pump while I was away to avoid getting engorged breasts).

5. Breastfeeding pillow: They are not necessary for single babies, as they often get in the way of getting a deep latch. With my eldest, I didn't have a breastfeeding pillow, but then I found it so, so great for breastfeeding my twins in the Rugby hold position (see page 89). When I first had the girls, I used one that looked like the number 3. They are very deep, so are great to help you not to have to lean forward. As the girls got older, I would just use lots of pillows or cushions from my bed or sofa, mainly to support underneath my arms.

6. Nipple shields: These were made originally for premature babies that have trouble latching due to their size and are something I used in both of my breastfeeding journeys. One of my nipples was slightly inverted

(funnily enough, it was the same nipple that cracked and I think this was because my eldest had trouble latching correctly) and so nipple shields helped me with this, and it was the same when I was breastfeeding my twins as they were so tiny, the shields really helped the girls to be able to latch.

I would always try first without, and after they latched, I would try to take the nipple shield off halfway to encourage them to latch without it. Be aware they come in different sizes and it's important you order the right size for your nipple so that it doesn't rub. It's also important to note that nipple shields, aka artificial nipples, can sometimes hinder your milk supply so I would advise a face-to-face with a lactation consultant before you try these out.

If you are looking to breastfeed exclusively, I would suggest putting money aside for a lactation consultant instead of buying bottles as a backup. If you are really wanting to continue breastfeeding, but you are struggling, getting some face-to face support is really important and I would recommend this to ANY mum thinking of stopping because they are struggling, but not wanting to stop breastfeeding yet. Invest your money in a lactation consultant and I'm sure you will have a much more positive breastfeeding journey because of it. Please go on to the LCGB website, and you can also check out credentials on the IBLCE website to ensure they have had the correct training. (see also Support, page 251).

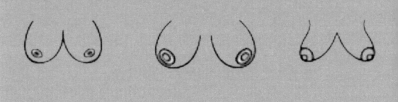

PART 4

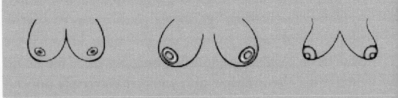

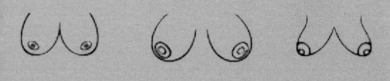

YOU'RE NOT ALONE

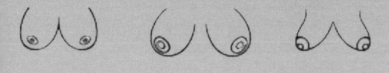

20

Breastfeeding After a Traumatic Birth

There are some things in life you just cannot plan for and giving birth is one of them. With Dakota, my eldest daughter, I attended hypnobirthing classes, I read all the books on labour and I wrote out the strictest birthing plan ever known to man. Unfortunately, it did not go to plan, but I still absolutely loved my birth. I ended up with medical interventions and instead of a planned home birth, I was chauffeur-driven to hospital by ambulance as my body just stopped dilating.

At the time when I was in labour, I was really upset that everything went out the window, but the moment I had my baby, I said it was the greatest experience I had ever had. I talk about my first birthing experience very positively. For some reason, at the time, I was really scared at the thought of giving birth in hospital, purely because I hadn't planned for that to happen, so I did not feel like my brain was mentally prepared for it.

As I said at the beginning, with my second pregnancy, I decided to try a different approach: I wanted to go with the flow, be open to changes that might happen. I had a basic plan, but wanted to be a lot more laid-back, as I knew however much I planned, my body would birth how it wanted to, something I had no control over. I ended up giving birth to Twin 1 (Tatum) naturally with forceps and Twin 2 (Blakely) ended up being an emergency C-section. After giving birth to my first twin, my cervix started closing. This was something I had no control over; I knew that it was a possibility, but this happens to such a small percentage of women[1]. For me, my experience with the twins was a traumatic one, for not just this reason but a number of different reasons, and even to this day, it's something I can still struggle to talk about.

At the time, I had so many emotions going through me and a whole world of thoughts flooding my head when they told me I couldn't have my second twin naturally. They sent my husband, mum and sister out of the room and in came a lot of people I had never seen before. It was scary to say the least. Even writing this now brings tears to my eyes. I knew it was important not to panic, to get the thoughts out of my head and just do what had to be done.

With my first pregnancy, I had done a hypnobirthing course and I had wanted to do it when I was pregnant with the twins but was told there was no point. Well, I strongly disagree! It had been three and a half years since I completed the course and straight away, I remember telling myself I needed to get into my hypnobirthing zone, especially when I was told I was going to have an

---

[1] www.nhs.uk/conditions/pregnancy-and-baby/giving-birth-to-twins/

emergency C-section for twin two. I became full of anxiety and I knew I needed to calm down and go with it to help this situation. I closed my eyes and started imagining a waterfall (this is what we were told to do all those years ago) and then I heard the sound of the water flowing, I really took myself to that place. Next thing I knew, my husband was back by my side and from what I can remember, I had given birth to my second twin.

After having a traumatic birth, your breastfeeding journey can go one of two ways. For me, I had a huge desire to regain some control. After I gave birth to both the girls, I had this very overwhelming urge that I just needed to breastfeed. I remember feeling like I wasn't a new mum of two beautiful daughters, but just a person lying on a bed in the middle of theatre, with lots of strangers around me and not 100 per cent sure of what went wrong and what was going on. I really needed to feel like I was a mum and get the instant connection that I had when I had given birth to my eldest. I needed to get everything back together again, physically. After giving birth to the girls, I felt like my body had failed me, so I needed my body to put things right and that was the start of our breastfeeding journey.

The other path you may go down, and please know this is in no way your fault if you feel this way, is that your body has already let you down, so how is it supposed to work in the right way now? How is it supposed to produce enough milk to feed your brand-new baby? How will it give them the correct nutrients? You may lose your confidence in yourself and in your body. Thousands of women a day give birth and yours has not gone to plan. After having a traumatic birth, learning a new skill like breastfeeding with a newborn baby can be very overwhelming – it can be overwhelming even after a straightforward birth. This is probably going to be the most physically and mentally demanding thing you will ever go through, so be completely kind to yourself. Many women birth babies, but each is unique, none of us have control of how our bodies birth, how long we might be in labour for, or if interventions will be needed.

A traumatic birth can lead to a delay in milk coming in due to large blood loss, but it's important to know that it is absolutely possible to still be able to breastfeed exclusively. What you must know is that it's not your fault at all if there's a delay in your milk coming in or if you lack the ability to be able to breastfeed, it's purely down to the situation, which has compromised your hormones that your body requires to promote breastfeeding. Please remember, as I've said above, this does not mean you will not be able to breastfeed – you will still be able to, but it's something to bear in mind and prepare yourself for, should this situation arrive.

It's important to know about the possible interventions that may arise in your labour, so you can make an informed decision. When we think about planning our births and labour, something you wouldn't normally think about is how the choices you make could affect your breastfeeding journey. The choices we make for our labour and birth are normally to help get us from

A to B. The medical professionals will suggest the decision they think is best for you and your baby, what they believe is the safest option, but ultimately the decision will always be yours.

If you do experience interventions, this doesn't mean that you cannot breastfeed. I just want to lay this out below so I can fully prepare you and let you know about the issues that may arise with certain interventions:

- Induction of labour – hormone drip
- Speed up labour – hormone drip
- Epidural
- IV (Intravenous) fluids
- Assisted birth
- C-section birth
- Mother and baby separation after birth.

In my last pregnancy, I had the hormone drip to speed up labour, an epidural, IV fluids, assisted birth with Twin 1 and emergency C-section with Twin 2. Although these things can have an impact at the start of your breastfeeding journey, it is also absolutely possible to be able to successfully breastfeed – you just need support, knowledge and determination.

Taking back power from a traumatic birth

I'm so lucky to have given birth to three healthy, happy babies, but I did have a traumatic birth with my twins. It's two and a half years on now and something I still struggle to talk about. I remember after giving birth to the girls being wheeled out of theatre into the recovery area. I had already had my first breastfeed with one of my twins, but I looked at my mum and sister who were waiting for me in recovery and I remember so clearly saying to them, 'I feel nothing like a mother, I do not feel like a mum at all.'

I want you to know, if you're reading this and you feel this way, then you are not alone, this is so normal. Traumatic births can affect you in ways you sometimes cannot explain or make sense of. Weirdly, sometimes I feel like I really want to relive my birth. I'm not really sure why, but I think maybe so I can take it all in and understand more. Maybe I feel like if I could live it again, I could somehow get some control back. But what I do know is that it's your birth and you're allowed to feel how you feel: your feelings are valid.

Speaking about my birth online was a huge step for me and something that really helped me understand what I had gone through. The girls were over one year old at the time and I felt like it was important to talk about their birth, for myself and for any other mums who may have been feeling the same as me. I will always remember someone's comment: 'Oh, I've heard about mums like you! Your birth didn't go to plan and all you want to do is moan about it.' I sat there and started questioning my feelings – was I being over the top? Maybe I shouldn't have shared this. I spoke to someone about it, said I felt selfish for being upset when I had given birth to three healthy babies, and they said to me, 'There will always be someone that has it worse than you have, but that does not make your experience less traumatic. Your feelings are real, you lived that, no one else.' And do you know what? I will never ever doubt or feel selfish for how I feel about it now.

Your birth is your story, it doesn't matter if your friends, cousins or aunty were in labour for six days, and you were only in labour for six hours. If you feel a certain way about your labour, no one else's experiences should take that away from you.

If you are struggling to deal with a traumatic birth, I would highly suggest speaking about it, maybe even writing your birth experience down on paper so it's not bottled up and you are getting it out there, and to seek out a therapist. You can get one for free through your GP, but you may have to wait. Or search online for someone privately with good reviews if you are able to afford it. I started seeing my therapist when the twins were two – I knew I had to see one and she has been worth her weight in gold!

Something else you can do is book a debrief session with the midwifery team. They will talk you through your notes and discuss why things happened the way they did, and will hopefully give you a little more understanding.

21

Hormones & Baby Blues

You may have heard of the term 'newborn bubble' – when you have given birth to your baby and it's nothing but you and your new arrival, the outside world just doesn't matter. You're in the thick of getting to know your child, getting to know their little signals, practising your breastfeeding positions, having lots of skin-to-skin. It's a wonderful place to be and I'm sure if someone could bottle up that feeling and sell it, they would be very rich.

Even in your newborn bubble, you will more than likely during the week after giving birth be affected by something known as the 'baby blues'. Your oestrogen and progesterone drop a lot after childbirth. These are hormones that are important for sexual and reproductive development in women and the amount of oestrogen and progesterone in your body will vary over your lifetime. So even with the new arrival of your little soulmate, the rapid drop in your hormone levels and chemical changes in your body are of course more than likely to affect you. Plus, you have just been through something so physically exhausting, childbirth, and will more than likely be very tired from round-the-clock feeds and nappy changes, and in general adjusting to this new life you are about to start.

It is overwhelming, and rightly so.

The good news is this should pass within a week or two. If you are wondering if you are experiencing baby blues, here's what to look out for:

1. Feeling emotional and tearful for no apparent reason
2. Anxious and restless
3. Overwhelmed and irrational
4. Low mood.

One thing you can do to make yourself feel better is sleep as much as you can. I know, this is nigh on impossible, especially with an influx of visitors and a baby needing to be fed through the night. Try and stop visitors coming over unless you trust them to look after your baby for a little while, have a break, lie with your baby and do nothing, try and nap while your baby naps, maybe get out of the house for a walk with your child in their pram or sling, get help from your partner or any other family and friends. The best thing to do if you are feeling low is to speak with the people you are closest to.

Could it be more than baby blues?

Even if you have gotten through the baby blues, of course you will still have tough days: maybe you can't stop your baby crying, or you're struggling with breastfeeding.

There may be days when you cry because you feel like you cannot cope. This is completely OK – remember you are having a complete lack of sleep and not enjoying a lot of self-care.

If you are worried about how you are feeling, there are some signs to look out for that mean you should maybe seek some extra help:

- Crying a lot
- Worrying about your baby's health and having intrusive thoughts
- Not being able to enjoy things you normally would or see happiness in things that would usually make you smile
- Loss of appetite
- Not being able to sleep
- Feeling like you want to harm yourself or your baby.

If you are feeling any of the above, please seek professional help. Go to your GP or health visitor. Ask them about support services in your area as they may be able to put you in touch with a counsellor or local support group. Meeting other women who are going through something similar to you can be so helpful and reassuring. Your mental health is so important to look after. You will be so busy running around and looking after your baby, don't forget to look after yourself in the process.

A lot of mums worry if they take anti-depressants that they will have to stop breastfeeding, but they are safe and you are able to continue to breastfeed. Please check out the website Breastfeeding Network's 'Drugs in breastmilk' page. Also speak with your doctor or health professional – tell them how you're feeling and your desire to continue breastfeeding.

Even if you are unsure about how you are truly feeling, speak to someone. A national support group that you can contact for advice is the Association for Post-Natal Illness (APNI): call the helpline on 0207 386 0868 (10am to 2pm, Monday to Friday) or email info@apni.org.

You are not alone.

Can breastfeeding affect your mental health?

Breastfeeding can help new mums' mental health. There was a study in 2014 with 10,000 mums that showed that mothers most at risk of post-natal depression were those who planned to breastfeed but were unable to – they were twice as likely to become depressed than the mums who decided they didn't want to breastfeed and so didn't.[1]

The importance of getting good breastfeeding support and knowledge to be able to succeed and breastfeed for your own mental health is clearly evident from this survey. It is incredibly important for a mum if their breastfeeding journey ends before they are ready to

---

[1] https://www.cam.ac.uk/research/news/breastfeeding-linked-to-lower-risk-of-postnatal-depression

stop; this is proven to mentally affect them. There is more research available on the UNICEF website that goes into this.

I wanted to breastfeed so much and felt such a lack of support when I needed it most, in hospital, surrounded by healthcare experts. After having my twins, going through a traumatic birth, I desperately wanted to breastfeed. If I had listened to the health-carers and done exactly what they had asked, I would not have breastfed. After I had my girls, I went to a lot of trouble to convince midwives that I could breastfeed. If I had not breastfed, I know this would have affected my my mental health ten times over, because successfully breastfeeding the twins was such a passion, want and need that had it been taken away from me before I was ready but due to lack of support, it would have been something that stayed with me forever.

My mental health after my second pregnancy

I know this is such a cliché, saying, 'It's OK to not be OK', but it's so true. Here, I want to share with you my own mental health struggles after having my twins.

The moment they both arrived in the world, everything went wrong. At first, they didn't arrive as planned and the birth was traumatic, so I was struggling very much with this. Then I tried to start my breastfeeding journey, which felt like a battle between me and my healthcare professionals, for them to actually respect my wishes of wanting to exclusively breastfeed the twins. This start to my breastfeeding journey with the twins is something that I couldn't even talk about until the girls were well over a year old.

We had four days in the hospital together, when they were first born. Then when the twins were six days old, we were back in hospital again for another stay, as both my girls couldn't regulate their temperatures and had to be put in an incubator. I think this was the moment I really significantly remember feeling so overwhelmed. I cannot describe the feeling, but I truly felt like I was drowning and nothing from the start of labour to this point was going right. I remember very clearly telling my husband the hospital were keeping both twins in to get them to regulate their temperatures, and even writing this now, I'm welling up completely involuntarily and my chest is tightening.

I felt like I had failed them – me, their mum – I couldn't even help them to stay warm. Obviously, my rational brain knows I did absolutely everything I could and it was completely out of my hands: they both had no fat on them and they were so tiny, they couldn't regulate their temperature just yet. But at the time, it felt like a stab to my heart. I was also completely torn because my eldest daughter, who was three then, had just had us back home for two nights and now her mum, dad and two new little sisters were off again together while she was left at home with her nan and grandad.

I felt so much guilt, I was completely overwhelmed; I just longed for us to be back home together as a family. I couldn't help but feel like I was being judged, that I was under pressure to perform as 'Mum'. I had to write down when the twins fed, how long for, and I remember feeling so nervous every time I was asked when they'd had their last feed. I was their mum but I felt like I was being vetted by the healthcare professionals. My grandad Cole Cole was dying at the time and I had a call one evening while we were still in hospital to say, 'I don't think he's going to make it until the morning.' I felt so torn, me and my grandad were so close, I had my two tiny babies lying next to me in an incubator and I couldn't leave them, and I couldn't be with him, by his side. I was completely anguished and mentally I felt broken.

Grandad Cole Cole made it through the night and carried on fighting. We were allowed to go back home after a few days once the twins started to be able to regulate their temperatures on their own. They were a week and a half old by this point and we only had a few days left of my husband Lewis being around before he went back to work. We hadn't spent any time as a family yet, on our own, bonding. Lewis was driving us back and forth every day, over half an hour away, there and back to see Grandad. It was so heartbreaking, watching him, my best friend, deteriorating every day in front of my eyes, but also trying to be happy when I was away from him and falling in love with my beautiful new babies and the new life I had brought into this world.

Around then, I started building up a wall around my emotions. I couldn't feel heartbreak for my grandad because I had to keep everything together to be able to parent my three children, so I ended up shutting off my feelings because I felt like I couldn't afford to feel anything. I knew I loved the twins, but I just didn't feel it – I felt numb and shut off. I remember feeling sick with worry that something was going to happen to them, because everything had been going wrong. I remember thinking to myself, this was the best way, don't feel anything, and then if something did happen, I would be able to handle it a lot better. I didn't want to see visitors, but I really wanted to establish breastfeeding with the girls, so we spent a lot of time in bed with lots of skin-to-skin and latching on. Also, I spent a lot of time on my own, trying to get to grips with becoming a mum of twins, but even with a lot of bonding I felt numb and closed off.

One day, I was on my way back from seeing Grandad and out of nowhere I started feeling really ill. I was dripping with sweat and I had the shakes and knew I had a temperature. It was mastitis. My doctor admitted me to the postnatal maternity ward and I was there on my own, waiting for Lewis to join us. That's when I got the phone call, four weeks to the day of giving birth to the twins, that my beautiful grandad had lost his fight. It was just me and the girls on our own, surrounded by lots of happy people that had just given birth.

I knew the time was coming, and it was such a relief he was no longer in pain, but my heart was broken. Completely and utterly broken. Luckily I was discharged and able to come home that day, which I needed, to be with Lewis and my three daughters together.

Two weeks later, we were blue-lighted back to the hospital as Blakely (Twin 2) had really bad bronchiolitis and was struggling to breathe. I thought that was it, after constantly worrying and imagining bad things were going to happen to the twins because everything had been going wrong. I questioned myself, thinking, was it my fault she was ill because I had been so scared something was going to happen? Was this my doing? Once we were in hospital, they told me Tatum couldn't stay with us as she wasn't admitted. I explained I was exclusively breastfeeding them both and I couldn't be separated from them, I completely broke down to the nurse and felt anxiety like I never had before. Thankfully they allowed Tatum to stay with us, and after a few days we were allowed back home.

I was mentally unwell and I didn't even realise. I was struggling with the girls, my feelings were numb and I was just going through the daily motions of life, from one day to the next. I felt like I was drowning on a daily basis, but, somehow, getting just enough air to keep on going. I didn't feel depressed in the sense I was really sad – I just did not feel happy, I didn't feel anything.

I had heard that twins got easier to handle from six months and I counted down the days. I wished the days away to myself, so I could get to that point and was then filled with guilt for wishing the days by. I felt like a terrible mum: how could I feel this way about my beautiful babies? I should have been enjoying every moment, taking it all in, and here I was wishing there was a fast-forward button. I remember breaking down to my mum and she said to me I was allowed to feel exactly how I felt and wishing their time away wasn't going to actually make it happen, so I had nothing to feel guilty about. It wasn't rocket science, but something definitely clicked in my head and eased my guilt.

Everything had a domino effect from the moment I had my traumatic birth. I had developed anxiety and one time I remember physically shaking so much, I couldn't pick the girls up. I couldn't speak about my birth to anyone. If anyone asked me how I was finding the girls, I would have to fight back tears and put on a brave face. You only have to look at my Instagram page to see that I hid all this very well. I spoke briefly at the time but nothing like the real truth, I was too scared to open up and not be able to actually handle the emotions I was feeling.

I knew I was struggling with losing my grandad, the traumatic birth and how much hard work the girls were, but I didn't truly appreciate how unhappy I was until I was happy again. The twins were one year and three months old, I was cleaning the kitchen and singing and dancing, and it was as if someone hit me over the head and it clicked: I was happy. How long had it been since I had felt that way? I hadn't sung away to myself since the moment the twins arrived. That was when my mental health changed, because I started acknowledging my feelings, grieving for my grandad, speaking and thinking about my birth. I was finally aware of my feelings.

I also decided to take my breastfeeding journey into my own hands when I found out another twin mum had gone through the same experience as me at the same hospital. When I read about her journey, it was like I was reading my own words and my heart broke for her. I was so angry that after I had complained about how I was treated, over a year on nothing had changed. I emailed the breastfeeding specialist at the hospital, I was crying and shaking as I was writing because I was so upset and annoyed that someone else was going to be affected like I was. After a few emails and a short time passing, I got a reply that they would change the training that their midwives have on mums wanting to breastfeed multiples. I felt a small triumph and in a weird way I had got some control back and had hopefully changed and helped future parents.

Don't get me wrong, I still have anxiety and I have seen a therapist and continue to see her on and off, but mainly now because I do not want to go backwards. I'm so proud of how I came out the other end from my mental ill health and that I can now speak openly about my troubles to hopefully be able to help someone else.

I didn't write all this down to sound depressing, or for sympathy, it's because I'm now strong enough to speak about it. Mental health problems are as real an illness as mastitis. I'm in no way ashamed of how I felt. It's important to know that anyone can go through it, at any time.

I was also affected by the start of my breastfeeding journey and my twins and I successfully breastfed for two years and three months. To some people, that might sound bizarre, but that's the thing with mental health: it's your mind, your story, your struggles, how you feel is how you feel, no one can take that away from you, or play it down.

IT'S OK TO NOT BE OK.

22

For Anxious Mums
by Anna Mathur

The post-natal weeks and months challenge mental health in so many ways. Whether you've jumped in with both feet into baby sensory classes, coffee socials and WhatsApp groups, or are finding solace on the sofa in a dressing gown, our experiences vary so much. As a psychotherapist and mum of three, I've got some tips and things for you to think about, so that you can ensure this time is as special as it can be.

- Check in with yourself. So many times, I ask a fellow mum what they feel or need. Pre-baby, this may not be something we need to give much thought to, as we have responded to our own needs without thinking much. However, when we suddenly become responsible for a baby, our attentions shift from our own feelings and needs, to theirs. Whilst this is natural, it's also vital that you are also asking yourself how you feel or what you need. Just because you have a baby doesn't mean you need to deprioritise your own feelings and needs; if anything, they need more focus than normal! How do you feel? What do you need? How might you take a small step to meet that need?

- Keep talking. Ensure that you are talking to at least two close friends or family members. So many of us have standard responses to being asked if we're OK. Regardless of how 'OK' you feel, it's good to encourage yourself to think and share about your emotions at this time so that, should you have a wobbly day or two (utterly normal by the way, it's human response to change!), you've already got people you feel comfortable talking to. I had a period of post-natal depression and anxiety after having my second baby. I found it so much easier to share my journey in a forum online initially. In time, this gave me the strength and confidence to speak to those in my life who could support me further.

- Monitor your moods. There is so much that will impact your moods at this time. From hormone fluctuations, sleep deprivation, and the fact so much has changed and been challenged in your life! No feeling is invalid. Try not to invalidate your moods by telling yourself you should or shouldn't feel a certain way. This is how we find ourselves sweeping emotions under the carpet, ready to trip us up later on, or find us crying them all out in a meltdown over a spilt cuppa. If you're having more low days than OK days, speak with your health visitor or GP so that they can monitor you. So many mums ask me whether they have baby blues, or a bit of post-natal depression. If you're even asking that question, you are deserving of support, regardless of how many boxes you tick!

- Mum guilt has become the norm. It sits heavily in our stomachs like a rock. Yet so much of it is unjustified and not about 'fault'. Guilt is there to prompt you, not to shame you. Next time you feel a wave of guilt for whatever reason, ask yourself why you feel guilty. What would you say to a friend who also felt guilty about this? Then bring in some words of kindness and compassion, in the way you would to a friend. Finally, what tweak might you make to ensure you aren't met with this wave of guilt again? Perhaps speaking about it to a friend, or visualising letting it go like a balloon. Unjustified guilt fuels critical internal dialogue and self-sabotage. We don't need more of that in our lives!

- Keep tabs on your internal dialogue. How are you speaking to yourself in the quiet of your mind? Are you kind and patient, or critical and cruel? Would you speak to a loved one or your baby in that way? If not, it's simply not good enough for you either! That's the truth of it. When you find yourself being critical, please try and bring in a kinder voice.

- It is so very common for anxious thoughts to spike when feeling tired, overwhelmed or hormonal. Next time you have an anxious or intrusive thought, count back from 100 in threes to distract your mind, and then use a simple breathing exercise to calm your body down from any fight or flight feelings (in for four, out for six x ten). Anxiety rises when we think about the unknowns.

— Now, don't cringe, but I'm going to mention self-care in a very non-cheesy way, I promise. Think of self-care as self-preservation. It's a vital cornerstone to good mental health but has been dangerously de-prioritised as an optional indulgence. Acts of self-care aren't just spa trips, but drinking enough water or addressing cruel internal dialogue. Self-care is asserting personal boundaries with overbearing relatives, making sure you eat lunch, and even going for a wee when you need one instead of hopping around the house. Take your space where you can, even if it means asking for someone to take the baby so that you can get some rest. It's not only good for self-esteem and mental health, but being kind to yourself is also an act of love towards those who love you!

I hope these tips are helpful. My book, *Mind Over Mother*, is jam-packed with more. I just want to say to you, you deserve for this experience to be a life-giving one, not a life-sapping one. You are worth support, as and when you need it, and you will not be a burden on the right people. Share your experiences and feelings with those who have historically been kind and supportive. Anxiety and worry are so common, but they need not rob you of a positive post-natal experience! There is so much more for you than that.

23

Physical Changes

If you would rather not read about sex, maybe skip the next few pages . . .

I am what you might call a bit of an open book (no pun intended!), so I wanted to tell you about my own experience of sex after giving birth and breastfeeding. I have a very healthy attitude towards sex! If I'm stressed with the girls then I'm probably over being touched by the end of the day and want some personal space. But then on the other hand I might just need to feel connected with my husband and be craving some intimacy. There really is no wrong or right. And each is completely normal.

After I gave birth to my eldest, the thought of having sex was NOT on my radar for a good while. I was told to avoid having sex in the first six weeks (this is advised to give yourself time to heal and to not put yourself at risk of having complications after giving birth), and at six weeks, was I ready to jump on my partner? No way, not a chance! I was absolutely exhausted; my daughter was in the middle of a growth spurt so cluster feeding like crazy and it was literally the last thing on my mind. I felt closer to my partner than ever after having our baby. It solidified our relationship and we had a deeper love and connection that wasn't there before, I strongly believe, but sex was not on my mind for a long while.

At around four months post-partum, I started feeling like I really wanted to be intimate again, but I tore during the birth and needed stitches, so I was petrified at the thought of having sex, even though I felt ready. I went to the doctors and got her to check my scars.[1] (I swore I'd been stitched up too tightly, but she told me it looked 'perfect'! What a compliment for my vagina after giving birth!)

Even though I was really nervous the first time after giving birth, I felt even closer and more connected to Lewis and the experience took our whole sex life to another level. I thought once you became a mum, that was it, your sex life was over. But for me, I felt like it was just beginning. You may not have this same feeling, and that is also normal! Sit down, speak to your partner and tell them how you feel, and if you have any worries or concerns, as it can be quite nerve-wracking the first time after giving birth.

There really is not a wrong or right time frame, it's completely up to how you feel. Mentally and physically,

---

[1] You'll come across a recurring piece of advice in this book – to always seek out a professional if you feel the need, or want to know more about a specific subject. That was one of the lessons I had to learn, that it's OK to reach out for help and doing so is the best thing for you.

you have gone through something major and we all heal at different rates. It's really important to wait until you are 100 per cent ready.

Breastfeeding can have an effect on your libido – after all, our hormones play a massive part in helping to produce milk in the first place. You may feel like you have no sex drive at all, you may feel like your sex drive is higher than before, or you may just feel the same. All of these feelings are completely normal. When I asked friends and followers how they felt about sex, breastfeeding and birth, I was inundated with messages from mums saying, 'I have been touched all day, my bed is for me to sleep in and have my own space.' Sometimes partners can find this difficult to understand as it's usually only one of you breastfeeding around the clock, so it's good to explain to them how you are feeling. There are so many other ways you can connect with each other: a nice meal, just the two of you or watching a film together, snuggling on the sofa. Just because you don't want to be physical doesn't mean you can't have an intimate relationship.

Vaginal dryness

Your oestrogen levels are lower than in those who aren't breastfeeding, so you may experience vaginal dryness. Something I would definitely recommend is water-based lubricant for any sexual activity! Do not feel embarrassed, this is most certainly normal, and if you don't feel comfortable picking up a bottle in store, then you can order some online.

Leaking milk

Something else you may not experience or know about is when you orgasm, your milk can leak out! When you breastfeed, you release oxytocin and the same thing happens when you orgasm. This is not something I experienced when I was having sex as a breastfeeding mum the first time around, but it was something that happened the second time around. It was just so unexpected, me and my husband both burst out laughing.

If this thought is something that makes you feel uncomfortable, speak with your partner beforehand and let him know that this could happen, or you could take a break from your nursing bra and wear some nice lingerie. A great way to stop the flow is to press onto your nipples for a few seconds.

How will I feel about my body?

The moment you become pregnant your body will go through so many changes. Some of these changes are temporary and some are not so temporary. You may get stretch marks (I got stretch marks in my bum crack – I mean, seriously, of all the places!). My ribcage expanded, especially after having the twins, which has not gone back to normal. My breasts are definitely looser, but I actually love how they are now. I grew up having no breasts at all, I used to wear socks in my bra when I would go out. Years before I had children, I had a fat transfer into my breasts, but I found they went back to normal. Since breastfeeding, I do not wear a bra and although my skin is looser, sagging is minimal and my breasts are a lot bigger.

I was taunted by a family member when I told them I would like to breastfeed my twins – she kept laughing hysterically and telling me my boobs were going to be down by my ankles. Considering they have fed my children for years, I love them and feel immensely proud of them: they fed, comforted and nurtured my three children!

I know many women who have never breastfed, who complain about how much their breasts have sagged after pregnancy. You are always told that it isn't breastfeeding that makes your boobs sag, it's pregnancy, but even I always found that hard to believe. But just from my own little bit of research among women I know, it's completely correct. I know some women choose not to breastfeed due to the worry of their breasts sagging, but this should not be a factor as pregnancy can cause breasts to sag and genetics play a huge part as well. Some women's breasts go back to normal and some don't; some stay larger, some shrink.

After breastfeeding, you will hopefully feel empowered by what your body has done and is still doing, because it's an absolutely remarkable thing. But sadly, of course some women may struggle with the changes their body has gone through. If this is you, then please know you are not alone. I think it's so easy to log onto social media and see lots of women preened to perfection, some may have even photoshopped their images, and to then end up feeling alone with your body changes and how you feel about them. Remember, everything you see on social media is normally someone's highlight reel, so you will never really know how they feel about their bodies. But there is a new fantastic movement online which is helping to change the way that we as a society see post-partum bodies: there are so many mum accounts showing their bodies in true form, unedited, all shapes and sizes. We are all normal, each and every woman, our shapes are different, the way our body changes is different, there is no right or wrong. Unfortunately, it is rammed down our throats to see, celebrities 'snapping back after birth' as the given and then those celebrities who don't have the trim, toned bodies are slammed in the press.

I have had the biggest body hang-up about the cellulite on the backs of my thighs. It's something I've always felt self-conscious of, especially after I became a mum for the second time around as my cellulite seemed to be worse than ever. We went on holiday to Florida when the twins were 18 months and the eldest was five. When we were lying around the swimming pool, I would get up with a towel wrapped firmly around me so no one could see my thighs. At the last minute I would quickly whip my towel off and jump in the swimming pool, hoping no one saw my thighs. A few days into the holiday, I thought to myself, *What the hell am I doing?* I have three beautiful daughters who look up to me and

I would be heartbroken if they behaved in the way I did. So, from that day, I ditched the towel. I did feel self-conscious at first, walking around the water park in just a swimsuit – I can't remember the last time I would have felt confident enough to do that, maybe when I was 18?

Do I love my cellulite now? No, but I appreciate this is my body, I am a woman and over 90 per cent of us have cellulite. I'm going to start embracing it, because I would love for my girls to grow up feeling completely comfortable in their own skin and know that they are normal, that we are all different and unique and still beautiful.

That really is the same after you give birth. I know some women, especially after a traumatic birth, or who are struggling to breastfeed, can resent their bodies and start picking holes in what they see as flaws. But they are not flaws because there's no such thing as the perfect body, this is just what the media portrays to you. After having Dakota, my body was the slimmest it had ever been, and after having the twins, I am now the largest I have ever been. Do I think for a second that I parent better, or my partner or children loved me more when I was slimmer? No way! There are things you can do to help change your mindset, starting with unfollowing people on social media who make you feel bad about yourself. Follow those who inspire you, follow this amazing movement of loving yourself, the body that made your baby, brought them into this world and then produced milk to keep them alive!

To close this chapter, here are the thoughts of my friend Kerri Northcott, founder of Coco + Indie (@life_with_ivycoco):

Nobody really tells you what your body goes through during pregnancy and how it changes after you've given birth. There is so much pressure to snap back to your pre-baby body and fit back into those jeans.

Why is this? Why do we put the pressure on ourselves? We just grew a human!

Our bodies grew and carried life and yet once we have birthed that life, we are thinking about getting into our old clothes. My body changed so much after giving birth to my daughter Ivy and I struggled so much. I wish I could go back in time and shake myself to get a grip.

Every diet you can think of, I did it. I was so self-conscious that before our first family holiday, I paid to have a treatment that would apparently melt fat. I was a size 12. I was ashamed of my stretch marks. I was riddled with anxiety at the thought of being seen in a bikini. I had just grown the most amazing little girl and was about to experience our first holiday together as a little family and this is where my head was, worrying about my post-baby body.

If you are currently struggling with accepting your post-baby body, I don't have a quick way to 'loving yourself, accepting your body'. We are all on our own journeys of self-acceptance. One day, I just thought, fuck this! My priorities in life have changed and my appearance ended up at the bottom of the pile.

Once Ivy started talking and repeating what we said, I think that was when the penny dropped. Would I ever want my little girl to feel she is not good enough because of her body? No way! Would I want her to ever comment or judge someone by their size? No. So I stopped dieting, I stopped talking about my body negatively and the word 'fat' is now seen as a swear word in this house. Stretch marks are now seen as love lines – they are little reminders of what my body did.

My only advice is next time you look at your body, or your child grabs your belly, and you notice the shimmer of a stretch mark, the new jiggle when you wiggle, remind yourself of how amazing your body is and look at what it created.

Remember the most important person that will love and look up to you will only ever want to see you happy and that they don't care if you fit into those jeans. In the grand scheme of things, life is just too bloody short not to eat the cake! Just make sure you do it out of sight of the kids, because we deserve to eat it in peace.

24

For The Bad Days

'I can't do this any more, I think I want to stop.'

This page is for the 'bad days' that will come, even if you are smashing this breastfeeding malarkey. Breastfeeding may be an instinct instilled in mums and babies, or it might not be. No matter how amazingly your journey is going, you will have days when you think, *Fuck, this is tough. Can I really carry on?* And I want you to know that is OK. You are completely allowed to feel this and you are 100 per cent not alone in feeling this. I would be very surprised to find a mum who has not had days like this.

If you are seriously considering stopping breastfeeding but you do not actually want to, and you are feeling this way because you are struggling, let me start by saying there is nothing wrong if you want to stop and formula feed, or maybe combi-feed for a little break. Whatever YOU want to do is important. I think your own mental health should come into consideration massively here. With the majority of mums I know who have stopped breastfeeding when they are not actually ready to have done so, it's more because they do not have the support or knowledge to carry on and end up regretting stopping. It's something that can mentally affect and play on your mind (*see* Chapter 21).That is why I honestly think it's so important to finish your breastfeeding journey because you truly want to and are ready to. If you make the decision to stop and you are ready, then great. And if you decide breastfeeding is not for you, once again, that is also great. It's so important to feed your babies how YOU want.

The mums I am speaking to in this section are those who may feel exhausted, or like they are struggling, or because they do not feel like they have any other choice but to stop, but don't want to. The first thing I would always tell myself when I was ready to throw in the towel (there were numerous occasions) was, 'Do not give up on a bad day, as tomorrow could be my best day'. I literally chanted this in my head, it was my mantra. What about if I gave up and tomorrow was the most amazing enjoyable day, because that was where I was looking to get to, not ending the journey completely. I didn't want to stop breastfeeding, but I did want to click my fingers and be at the amazing part. Getting there is tough, but I'm so glad I stuck with it through the dark days, and the only thing that kept me going was sheer determination (and also the motivation to prove everyone wrong that I could exclusively breastfeed twins!).

Turn to your support network, be it a Facebook breastfeeding group or your family or friends. Tell them exactly how you are feeling: sad that you do not want to stop breastfeeding, but like you have no other choice. Hopefully, you will have support and encouragement, or some friendly advice, and it might just be the little push you need to get over the hurdle. A problem shared is a problem halved, after all.

I mention this a lot, but I encourage you to speak with a lactation consultant. Maybe your struggle has got you doubting your ability to breastfeed your baby. If this is how you are feeling, then a lactation consultant will be able to give you their expert advice and knowledge to get you to feel more confident and maybe able to continue, if that's what you want (*see also* Support, 251).

Reasons why you are thinking of stopping:

'I'm not producing enough milk'

The chances are you've not been informed about cluster feeding and growth spurts. Please study Chapter 4, pages 67–75.

'My nipples are sore'

Has anyone looked at your latch and positioning, or checked your baby for tongue-tie? Watch YouTube videos on latching and positioning and re-read Chapter 5, pages 77–80, and Chapter 10, pages 113 and 119.

'Because I feel like I have no support!'

Have you tried a local breastfeeding group? Have you joined a breastfeeding Facebook group? Please re-read the Support section, pages 249–53.

If any of the above reasons are why you're thinking about ending your breastfeeding journey, please read over the chapters I recommend again and if you can afford it, pay a lactation consultant for face-to-face support. There are also breastfeeding charities you can call, who will be able to help you (see Support, page 249).

If you are thinking of stopping breastfeeding not because of any of the reasons above, but because you are truly ready to finish, then please read Chapter 12, pages 127–130 first.

25

What 'They' Don't Tell You

The start of this sentence is one I hear very often:

'They don't tell you it can hurt'
'They don't tell you how unnatural it can feel'
'They don't tell you babies have growth spurts'
'They don't tell you how to latch'
'They don't tell you they want to be on my boob all the time'
'They don't tell you . . .'

There is so much information not given to new mums and I'm not sure who the blame lies with. Should it be discussed when you're going through your checks when you're pregnant? Or on the ward after you give birth? You would think you would learn the ins and outs of breastfeeding in your antenatal classes, but that mainly surrounds your labour and giving birth.

Hopefully your midwife that you see while you are pregnant, or the team on the postnatal ward, can help you and give invaluable knowledge and advice, but what if they don't? What then? From my own personal experiences and speaking with so many mums, unfortunately more women are thrown in the deep end and left to figure it out. Now, we are also less likely to be surrounded by family and friends who have or who are also breastfeeding. We don't always have friends or family nearby and even if we do, often they haven't breastfed their babies. This makes it harder as we are much less likely to have our village and 'it takes a village to raise a child'.

When you are a new mum and do not know what you are doing, remember that your newborn baby has never done it before either! It can definitely feel like the most unnatural, alien feeling. It's completely fine and OK to feel this way: you are not the first and only person to feel this, and you will not be the last, so do not beat yourself up about feeling this way.

I think patience is key for success. If you want to breastfeed, but you don't feel like it is working for you, then reach out to a lactation consultant (*please see* Support), or call the National Breastfeeding Helpline on 0300 100 0212 – they may just provide you with the inspiration to keep at it a little longer, or give you some information to help the experience and make it all come together. It doesn't take long for you and your baby to become pros at breastfeeding. You could be a dab hand at it straight away, but it might take a little longer and with a bit of help, you can keep going for however long you want. No way is right or wrong – if you have set yourself a goal for how long to breastfeed one way won't make you reach it quicker, it will just be a different journey!

26

Real Mums, Real Stories

What's more inspiring than real mums' stories? I wanted each story to be different, I wanted you to see that there is hardship, but it pays off. I wanted each one to be unique and individual from the next.

Honestly, I feel so honoured to be able to share with you these stories. I read through them with tears in my eyes, goose bumps on my arms, and I felt truly inspired by the hurdles these women encountered and the choices they made. I could not feel prouder of this chapter if I tried! Each story proves the theory that breastfeeding is 90 per cent determination and 10 per cent milk!

* * *

Laura Wilton

In 2010, I was diagnosed with cervical cancer, two months before my wedding day and five months after getting the dreadful news of my mum's diagnosis of bowel cancer. At 24, you feel untouchable with the world at your feet, planning your future life, weddings and babies. To say this had a devastating impact would be an understatement. In that moment, being in the consultant's office and being given this life-changing news, your life, present, past and future, flashes before you. I remember the consultant saying, 'Most people's question at this point is, "Am I going to die?"' But this was not the question I wanted to immediately know the answer to: I wanted to know if I was going to be able to have a baby. I always knew that I wanted to have children. I was always going to be a mother, and from a young age I would breastfeed my dollies – a running joke in our family that was brought up on numerous occasions for years.

So, I embarked on the recommended treatment plan – initially surgery to preserve my fertility. I travelled to London from Devon the day after our wedding for a radical trachelectomy. Unfortunately, this was not successful and cancerous cells were found in the borders of my cervix. The next stage of treatment, radiotherapy and chemotherapy, would result in loss of fertility. Prior to eradicating my fertility, we were given the option to have eggs harvested and embryos made, which of course we jumped at. My husband and I were extremely fertile and thankfully, we were able to create lots of embryos to be frozen and one day potentially be a biological child.

Fast forward to 2017: unfortunately, we lost my mum in the November of 2010, but I had kicked cancer's ass. Following successful curative cancer treatment and a number of years trying to rebuild our lives, we found a brilliant, wonderful, selfless human and her family, who were willing to go above and beyond for two strangers and become our surrogate. I still pinch myself at just how lucky we were to meet such amazing people, there really are no words or ways to repay someone for doing something like that for you. Even more incredible luck was to follow and after our first attempt at embryo transfer, we received a big fat positive pregnancy test.

By then I had heard about inducing lactation and began to undertake research. I found a dedicated social media group and read through numerous protocols on how to artificially trick your body into producing milk. I talked to other mothers who had successfully induced lactation and breastfed their babies for differing lengths of times and all recommended *Breastfeeding Without Birthing* by Alyssa Schnell, and this book became my bible.

I followed the Newman-Goldfarb Protocols, which is a medical approach, as I felt due to hormonal changes as a result of chemo and radiotherapy, my body might not respond without a kickstart. As soon as we got the positive pregnancy test, I began by taking a birth control pill alongside a herbal supplement. It seemed bizarre taking the pill not to prevent having a baby, but in order to be able to provide for one. Six weeks prior to the birth, I began to pump or hand express every three to four hours, day and night, stopping the birth control pill and taking domperidone (an anti-sickness medicine) alongside herbal supplements. Getting my GP on board with the prescription of domperidone was the trickiest bit of all of this as it's not licensed for breastfeeding purposes, just a happy side effect of the medication. The herbal supplements I purchased from a local health food shop. I tirelessly pumped every three to four hours and that ecstatic moment when I got the first drop of milk was immense and I was able to store the expressed milk to use as top-up.

We were present at the birth of our beautiful baby girl and she was immediately placed on me for skin-to-skin and within a matter of minutes, she was on the boob. Wow, that feeling, the closeness and powerful bond, there's nothing else like it! For me, all that hard work of inducing lactation was worth it for that one moment, feeling like I was finally a mother.

She latched magnificently and fed well, it was all so natural. When I set about this process my initial goal was to be able to produce enough milk for that one feed and believe me, it would have been worthwhile for that moment, but we continued on: days became weeks, weeks become months. Mindful and worried about the amount of milk and whether there was a limit to the amount I'd be able to produce, I introduced a supplemental nursing system. We used expressed breast milk in the bottle that you wear round your neck with a small tube taped at the nipple to provide extra milk while being breastfed. This was a fiddly job but worked well once in place and gave me peace of mind that she was getting enough milk.

I breastfed our baby girl for three months in total for her main source of milk before introducing a bottle. If someone had told me I'd have been able to achieve this at the beginning, I wouldn't have believed them. I'm extremely proud of this achievement and so grateful to have been able to experience breastfeeding.[1]

Kirsty Alexander

'It may affect your ability to breastfeed' was something that has always stuck very clearly in my mind from the breast surgery I had when I was younger. My consultant had explained about severed milk ducts and trauma to my breast tissue that would cause potential complications and although I wasn't nearly ready to start a family, I had always imagined having babies and being able to breastfeed.

It wasn't until I first found out that I was pregnant that I started to panic about whether I would be 'good enough' and able to breastfeed my baby. But I remember seeing that very first tiny drop of colostrum in the shower at around 37.5 weeks and suddenly a glimmer of hope was there for my breastfeeding journey. I think that's where my determination to breastfeed started; however I definitely didn't have the realisation at that point of how hard it would be.

---

[1] Schnell, A. (2013) *Breastfeeding Without Birthing. A Breastfeeding Guide for Mothers Through Adoption, Surrogacy, and other special circumstances.* Praeclarus Press: Texas

When my eldest, Bonnie, was born, it was the most magical moment I'd ever experienced, but having to have a C-section meant that even from the moment she was born, I was already being told that 'combi-feeding with formula top-ups may be the best thing under the circumstances', and from that point, I remember feeling very much as though what I was so desperate to achieve for myself and my baby wasn't necessarily at the fore-front of every medical staff's mind.

I was lucky enough to have a great deal of support from family and friends but even when my milk was coming in around day 5, I remember calling the hospital in tears of panic because my breasts were so hard that Bonnie was struggling to latch. At the time I was told by the staff that if I couldn't get my milk flowing and get her to latch, I'd need to top-up with formula. The only advice was to have a hot shower. I felt very scared and unsupported and it wasn't until my next midwife visit that I was given some reassurance about the success we'd made with my milk levels and Bonnie's latch. Although I was able to breastfeed Bonnie, I struggled to get the levels of milk that she needed to keep her weight up and mainly fed from one breast while the other only produced a small amount of milk. I felt like I'd failed her in a way and rather than celebrating my breastfeeding journey, I definitely felt a lot of guilt around it and not being 'enough'.

When I found out I was lucky enough to be pregnant for a second time, and even more lucky that it was a multiple pregnancy (I was having triplets), that little twang of guilt around 'not being enough' immediately came back to me: How was I going to feed multiple babies when I struggled so much to solely feed Bonnie, surely one good boob wasn't going to cut it this time? I was also advised very early on at my booking-in appointment that I shouldn't get my heart set on solely breastfeeding as it would be very challenging with multiples – something I already realised, but still wanted to try. Fortunately, I had the most amazing midwife who supported me throughout and although I had a very traumatic and heartbreaking pregnancy with the loss of one of our precious triplets, Dotty, I was over the moon to give birth via a second C-section to a perfectly healthy Delilah and Wilfred, who needed no special care and were allowed straight into my arms.

I was able to get them both latched as soon as we went into the recovery room and had our magical first feed. After being tested, I was told that Delilah had slightly low blood sugar and advised to immediately top her up with formula. Looking back, I wish I'd insisted on the support of the feeding team but I was so worried about my baby's wellbeing that I agreed to give her formula. She was then re-tested and her levels had come up so significantly that they told me the low reading may have been a misread and that the machines were very temperamental – very frustrating news!

I breastfed with the support of the feeding team throughout my hospital stay, and they were amazing, helping me to manually express, supporting in keeping my sleepy babies awake, etc., but there weren't enough of them and they were completely run off their feet. At times I'd call for help with latch or positioning for tandem feeding Delilah and Wilf and we'd be told there was no one around and they'd send them as soon as they were free. Sometimes they'd make it to us, sometimes they wouldn't. We even stayed in an extra night purely for feeding support and on that evening, we didn't get a single visit despite our constant bell presses. It wasn't because they didn't care, because they really did, it was because they just didn't have the levels of staff to support everyone who needed it. I feel that if all midwives had feeding training for both single and multiple births then the levels of support would be hugely increased and mummies like me could feel that extra bit of confidence at the start of their breastfeeding journeys.

My own midwife Nikki and two wonderful ladies from the feeding team, Debbie and Louise, continued to be amazing when we left the hospital and supported me with everything I wanted to achieve for our journey. I also had the most wonderful support and advice from Chantelle and as a result of her beautifully kind and caring nature and her passion for breastfeeding, I had a pumping schedule, a 'switching' schedule to make sure that Delilah and Wilf got adequate time on my 'good' breast, breast milk cookies, supplements – you name it, I did it! Despite my efforts and the amazing support from Chantelle and my midwife, the babies still needed two formula top-ups a day, something I still feel a little disappointed with myself about, but I know I shouldn't! I should definitely be proud and luckily, I've been told that by so many people, including a lactation consultant, who I also decided to seek advice from to make sure I was doing all I could for my babies.

Feeding my three babies was hard work and feeding them mainly from one breast was even harder – it was draining, exhausting and completely overwhelming, but more than all of that, it was amazing! For me there was nothing more heart-warming than breastfeeding my babies and although there was definitely relief when I decided to end our journey, I definitely miss it and will always treasure that last time for each of them.

Rose Finneron

I breastfed my daughter for a year with no real issues so I knew when I became pregnant with my son that I would like to breastfeed him too. Unfortunately, things weren't so straightforward with him. I had a terrible pregnancy which resulted in my son being born prematurely at 27 weeks. He was born via emergency C-section under general anaesthetic. I was very unwell and sadly, I didn't see him for 14 hours after he was born. Even then, I could only touch my tiny 3lb boy through the doors of the incubator in Intensive Care.

I was informed straight away that babies born as prematurely as my son should not have anything other than breast milk as their tummies are just too sensitive for formula milk and as they have missed out on the antibodies passed through the placenta during the third trimester of pregnancy, it was so important he had my breast milk. I started expressing every two hours the day after he was born. It was such hard work, but it really got me through a terrible time as I felt like I was actually doing something to help him and it was the only way I really felt involved in his care.

Over a week later, I could finally hold my son. The nurses tube-fed him tiny amounts of breast milk and I could only hold him once a day if he was stable. I spoke to them about the possibility of me breastfeeding and most said to me that the majority of mums end up bottle feeding as premature babies get too tired and it can be really difficult to get a good latch with oxygen and feeding tubes in the way.

Despite his medical issues, I still had a strong desire to feed my son. At 31 weeks' gestation, I noticed my son rooting [turning his head] so I put him to the breast and to the nurses' surprise, he latched on and attempted to feed. It wasn't for long and he didn't have a perfect latch, but my tiny boy was learning what to do. I did this every day until finally he was needing fewer and fewer tube feeds. After 70 days in NICU, my boy came home on oxygen and exclusively breastfeeding.

My son is now 18 months old and we are still continuing our breastfeeding journey. He has chronic lung disease through prematurity – he spent eight months on home oxygen and can really suffer with his chest, especially during cold and flu season. The antibodies he receives through my breast milk help him fight off these bugs I think much quicker than his body would be able to without.

I love so much about breastfeeding! I'm amazed by the science of it, how it protects our babies and the bond it creates between a mother and baby – this was so important to me as I missed out on so much bonding time. My advice to any mum who wants to breastfeed would be to trust your body. If in doubt, offer the breast. Don't feel concerned about the frequency of feedings as it's completely normal for a newborn to want to feed regularly. It gets easier!

Lynsey Thompson

With my first son, I had no knowledge, no face-to-face support and honestly, no idea about breastfeeding a baby! So, when I was pregnant with my second, I joined every breastfeeding group, read every article and got clued up on anything and everything related to breastfeeding. We had a great start – he was born and within minutes was rooting. The midwives at the hospital were amazing at helping me with getting a good latch and once we felt like he was established breastfeeding, we got to go home.

On day 3, the pain throughout a feed would ease but somewhere along the way we had gotten a bad latch, and boom, my nipples were cracked! I couldn't bear anything touching my boobs so whenever I could, I'd lather on nipple cream and stay topless. Fast forward to day 6 and my right boob was itchy, red and shiny. The pain during a feed was no longer sore from my nipples but it had changed to a burning pain. It was like being stabbed through my back and out my nipple every single feed. I would cry when I knew he wanted feeding from that side. My good boob at this time was still cracked too, so any feed was painful and newborns like to feed a lot!

The morning of him being one week old, we had our midwife visit. The great news was that he was back to birth weight in just a week – all from my boobs! It was that pat on the back I needed to know that although I was feeling rubbish, he was thriving. The bad news was I had a womb infection, thrush in my boob, mastitis and a bacterial infection in the cracks of my nipples. They were badly infected. I ended up having to pump my right boob as it was so bad, he refused to latch on and then I couldn't store the milk because of the thrush, so if he wasn't cup-fed the milk while it was fresh, then down the drain it went.

At this point, I felt very overwhelmed. I felt like the baby blues were just not going away and I was scared of feeding him because of the pain. I made the decision to introduce a bottle and see how we went from there. Life kind of took over and with a poorly toddler with a winter bug, four infections and then a potentially retained placenta, I decided to put him onto bottles with expressed breast milk and formula when I didn't have anything expressed. It really broke me inside because I knew that this wasn't how I wanted to feed.

Three weeks later, I hadn't expressed for just over two weeks, I had stopped feeling full and leaking, and my boobs were healing. He still rooted for me, always looking to latch, and one morning, he was so upset at getting his nappy changed, I popped him in my onesie to do some skin-to-skin to calm him while we waited for the health visitor, and he latched on. I didn't know if getting back to breastfeeding could even be done but I knew that we needed a second chance at it.

The health visitor came in and I told her that I needed help getting back to breastfeeding. Admittedly, I still felt terrified but I knew with the right help, I could do it. We got face-to-face support from the infant feeding coordinator, expressed, did skin-to-skin and let him feed basically 24/7 to get my supply back up. It wasn't easy to work out how to do it, no one I knew could really advise on when to ditch the bottles and go back to full boob. I decided to give him as much boob as he wanted, then a 2oz bottle. After about a week I was shattered – feeding all the time, looking after a toddler and having to deal with bottles too – so one night, I went to bed and decided that I'd see how he was with no bottles and since then, we never looked back. His weight was great, plenty of wet and dirty nappies and he was content so I felt confident enough to go for it. I still had some cracked nipples that were nearly healed but not quite there, so my friend recommended Silverette Cups for healing them and it worked.

Getting back to exclusive breastfeeding was not easy but it can definitely be done. I really wish I hadn't stopped for those few weeks and had sought more face-to-face help and tried different healing methods and got our latch checked, but now we are at 13 months breastfeeding and I plan to let him self-wean when he's ready. I wish I could go back in time and tell myself then what I know now and that it'll all work out. After weeks of worrying about pace feeding, bottle preference and how his daddy will bond, eventually I ended up with a 'bottle-refusing, boob-obsessed baby' who shouts 'Daddy!' all day long and smiles the second he sees him.

Jodie Bacon

Throughout my pregnancy with my son Freddy we knew there were going to be a lot of unanswered questions. We already knew he had Down's syndrome and a lot of other complications and also that he would need to have heart surgery not long after being born, but since I already had a two-year-old girl that I had successfully breastfed for 11 months, feeding, ironically, wasn't one of the things that concerned me.

When Freddy was born by caesarean section three weeks early he was taken straight down to the NICU unit and given a feeding tube as standard procedure but it later came about that his suckle reflex was very weak and so my expressing journey began! Every day, every two hours, I would express milk for him to be fed through a feeding tube. Freddy was only 4lb when born, and with the possibility of at least one operation on the horizon, we knew he not only had to gain weight, but we had to be confident in feeding him this way.

The pump soon became my close companion! It wasn't what I had thought feeding my baby boy would be like (nothing like the blissful newborn days that I experienced with my daughter), instead a rather noisy hospital-grade breast pump and picture of Freddy to try and help the milk flow. Then, once it was feeding time, we would hold the syringe full of my breast milk up and connect it to his tube and it would gradually flow through. We did this every two hours without fail, day and night. Freddy didn't really cry so we would set alarms to wake up. The amount of times we nodded off and woke up covered in breast milk as we'd dropped the syringe on ourselves – and wasted precious breast milk! Oh, and of course, there's the joy that was mastitis – just what you need when you've had a C-section and are spending day and night on a NICU ward!

But even through all that, I knew I was doing my absolute best for my boy. As I couldn't hold him, it made me feel closer to him, like our special bond was even that little bit more special. After six weeks of breastfeeding, the doctors decided he needed to gain weight faster, so they put Freddy on high-calorie milk, so my breastfeeding time with him had come to an end. But I'm so pleased he got the best milk he could get for those six weeks.

Ida Maria

When we first found out we were expecting triplets, I was only six weeks pregnant and we were in a state of shock. With three children already, no intentions of having more, a tight budget and three C-sections in my backpack, the thought alone of growing three babies in my womb was scary. Bringing them into the family and being able to provide for them was even scarier. Not long after, we accepted the fact that three little lives had chosen to come into our family and then all the real worries began. How would we take care of them? Where would they sleep? How do I feed them? *Feed them?* Is it even possible to breastfeed three babies?

With my single babies, breastfeeding had been very natural and easy for me. It is very convenient, always having food on tap. Through the night being close to my baby, hearing them breathe and their heartbeat, reacting on the slightest sign of discomfort and being able to nurse them back to sleep, it is so calm and safe. That was the only way I knew, but I just couldn't see that picture with three babies.

I started searching the internet for breastfeeding triplets – in Danish as I live in Denmark – no luck. When I asked in Facebook groups for multiples, I was kindly told that it was fine to use formula. People around me said that it wasn't possible to breastfeed triplets. My mother, my mother-in-law, friends and strangers all said: 'Wow, triplets! But then you can't breastfeed . . .' I read about the necessity of bottle-feeding triplets by a schedule. Either waking them all up at a certain time or when one wakes up – 'then you need to wake up the others so they stay on the schedule'.

It just didn't feel right for me – nor my husband – the fact that someone told us what we had to do, it was like we had no choice in how to take care of our own babies. Already having three kids, we knew how we wanted to parent. We knew how we liked to do our feeds, sleeping, routines, etc. We knew what felt right for us. I was devastated that we might not be able to parent our triplets the way we had parented all of our singletons.

When I was 14 weeks into my triplet pregnancy, I got in contact with a La Leche League leader, who sent me three articles telling stories of triplet mums breastfeeding exclusively. It was late in the evening when I started reading their stories. Tears went down my face as I told my husband that it could be done. It was actually possible to just continue as we were used to – well, with three babies! It gave me my courage back, just knowing there were other mums like me out there who actually had done what I wanted to do, even though everyone around me told me I couldn't. I found a book saying that wet nurses in the old days could provide milk for six babies – hey, then I could certainly do three! I even found a Danish triplet mum who had breastfed her babies for five months. Soon I had all the proof I needed to believe in myself.

The next step was to figure out HOW to do it. There are definitely some math issues when you have three babies and two boobs! The most commonly suggested thing was to breastfeed two and give the third one a bottle and still keep the babies on a strict schedule. I wasn't keen on the schedule part – I had been used to feeding a baby when they were hungry and I wanted to keep it that way. Then I found another story that made me cry again. A triplet mum feeding one baby at the time – no bottles, co-sleeping, carrying babies in slings, attachment parenting in every way. She became my heroine. And that became my No.1 goal: to simply feed one baby at a time.

Feeding them individually would give me the quality one-on-one time with each baby that I wanted, it would make me able to go out of the house not worrying about bringing any bottles or pump, or cleaning them for that matter. I would be able to breastfeed lying down at night as I was used to and best of all, it would help keep my supply up. I was all in! But it turned out to be a bit different than we had hoped for. Our babies chose to arrive at 28 weeks. My waters suddenly broke half an hour after a check-up ultrasound showing that everything was perfect. A long and scary day at the hospital ended up with an emergency C-section at 2am and suddenly I was sitting with a breast pump alone in my own room, knowing my three little babies were two floors below in NICU – each in their own incubator with lots of wires and tubes. The staff told me to pump every three hours with a six-hour break at night.

Being pregnant with triplets, I was prepared for a preterm birth, though I had been sure that it wouldn't happen to me. I knew I was able to pump milk, I knew how to hand express and I was certain that I needed to pump more frequently than every three hours.

The first few days I could only hand express and I brought tiny measure cups with drops of colostrum for the feeding times and had to choose which baby to give my milk, the others would get donor milk. I used as much time as possible to have skin-to-skin with my babies. The hospital recommended two hours a day, which was hard enough having two babies in one room and one in another room. I pumped every two hours when possible and every three at night. My milk came in (as usual) on the third day and my supply was going up[2].

After three weeks of pumping and tube feeding, a nurse asked me if I wanted to try to put the babies on my breast. I shouldn't expect them to latch, but just let them be there. All three of them latched beautifully but weren't yet able to transfer milk. It took many weeks of training. I was determined to let the babies learn to breastfeed before any of them would have a bottle – even though the staff offered several times to get me

---

[2] In Denmark, parents are able to stay at the hospital when their baby is in NICU.

one, because 'that's how mums usually feed the third baby'. I told them I wanted to do this my own way and they respected my decision. The staff were amazing at all times, but with only around ten sets of triplets in Denmark a year, no one really knows that much about breastfeeding triplets. Even my family and friends who were originally negative were supportive after I told them that was the way I wanted to do this.

We had a four-week homestay before the babies were discharged from the hospital at week 38. At that time all I did was breastfeed. I had to weigh each one before and after breastfeeding to see how much milk they had transferred and then supplement with the rest in the NG tube. After doing that times three, I had to pump. Then I had an hour before the next feeding session.

It is crazy to think about it now, and there is no way I could have done it without my husband staying home on perinatal leave, supporting me and taking good care of our three older children. At that time, they were two, four and six years old and they were helping to change diapers [nappies] and pouring milk in the tubes when they wanted. They were very understanding that I had to feed the babies. All of us worked together to take care of them and each other. Even our community helped out by bringing food.

Until they were ten months, I exclusively breastfed, on-demand feeding, one baby at a time – all the time. I tried double feeding, but it made me feel trapped. With one baby, I can still cuddle the others, I can hug my big kids and I can get my coffee cup. No doubt it's hard work and it is definitely the craziest thing I have ever done. But I'm SO glad I didn't listen to the 'Dream Stealers' – I did what felt right for ME to do – and I still do.

Our triplet girls, Scarlett, Eleanor and Kendra, are now 20 months and we still breastfeed in the evening and night, and sometimes in between.

Lacey Smith

I am mummy to 20-month-old Henry, who I breastfed for 18 months, and a midwife. I think people just assumed when I had Henry that I would breastfeed because of my job and that I would take to it like a duck to water because I knew everything about it and helped women to do it on a daily basis. Well, everyone was wrong!

Firstly, I had actually planned to bottle feed because I was never that bothered about breast or bottle. Secondly, I took to it more like a duck to outer space. It was really hard.

I had a gruelling induction of labour, resulting in an emergency caesarean section, where I lost more blood than my body was happy with. I was so off my face on drugs afterwards that Henry's first few feeds were formula. I was in no fit state to breastfeed him, and as I mentioned before, I hadn't actually intended to do so. Then, when the ward visiting time finished and my husband was kicked out (even midwives don't get visiting time special treatment), I was left on my own with Henry and too embarrassed to keep buzzing, asking for some-one to sort out a bottle for me. I didn't want my col-leagues to think I was one of those buzzer-happy nui-sances, so when he was hungry, I took my knowledge of breastfeeding and put him on my boob. It was fine. No amazing rush of emotions over how wonderful feed-ing my newborn like this was. It was just fine. He then went to sleep and so did I. For about two hours anyway, before I did it all over again!

When my husband rocked up in the morning, I told him about breastfeeding and said I might just carry on for a while because it's easy (famous last words) and saves us faffing with sterilising and making up bottles. Just until I'm recovered from the operation, then I'll stop. Over the next few weeks my beginner's luck soon caught up with me. My nipples quickly started to get sore and I couldn't work out why when his attachment was perfect. He was diagnosed with a tongue-tie. Only a small one, but every feed felt like his gums had been replaced with razor blades. I'd spend the entire feed with my toes curled up, crying in pain. Then because he wasn't draining my breasts fully, I wound up with mastitis, which got so bad, I was readmitted and put on a sepsis care bundle. Plus, because he wasn't draining my breasts and was only getting the lighter foremilk, it exacerbated his reflux. I look back now and I wonder why I put myself through it. It honestly was awful; there was nothing wonderful and loving about it. It was pain-ful and exhausting!

But I did it because after having Henry, I felt like a failure. I cried all the time. I was so upset that I was induced and had a section. Even as a midwife, with everything I know and what I counsel women in all the time, I felt like my body failed at doing the one thing it was born to do: it failed to go into labour and then I failed to push a baby out. My mental health really suffered and I hid it well. The only people who saw my breakdowns behind closed doors were my husband and two midwife friends. Even now, almost two years on, I struggle to talk about my birth without crying. So, after this, I felt like I had to prove to myself that my body was able to do something it was born to do – I had to breastfeed!

Once I got rid of the mastitis and got Henry's tongue-tie snipped, I thought that would be the end of my problems. I was two weeks post-natal by this point and things were looking up. Then came cluster feeding. Sometimes Henry would suck at my boobs for over an hour! Every time I took him off, he would scream and nothing else would settle him except my boobs. I used to dread going out in case he had one of these spells, so I didn't go out, which didn't help my mental health in hindsight.

I stuck with it because of a few people – Facebook support groups, my Trust's infant feeding specialist midwife (who runs a Facebook group for women at my Trust to give them the same support and advice) and the author of this book! These people gave me the most incredible support and advice. I used to text Chantelle ALL THE TIME. In despair, questioning why everyone else made it look so easy, reflux problems, not sleeping, ranting about people telling me how to feed my child . . .

After listening to Chantelle's advice, I made it to six weeks and she was right: things did get easier. The growth spurt was exactly as relentless as she warned me. But afterwards Henry just sort of got himself into a slight routine. The cluster feeding finished. I no longer had to apply the methods we teach women anymore, to think about nose to nipple, nice straight line and all that jazz. Henry would go on if I was doing a handstand! He was an established breast feeder and my supply finally calmed down. At that point, I was so proud of myself for persevering and so glad I didn't give up, because Chantelle was right, I would have regretted it.

After that, breastfeeding became like a drug and a third parent. If Henry was tired, teething, bumped his head, I could just put him on my boob and make everything better for him. After Henry's first birthday I had so many people asking if I was going to stop now. Some gave me funny looks when I said no. We're both still enjoying it. I honestly don't understand it. My child, my body, my choice. Then shortly after he turned 18 months old, he quickly lost interest in breastfeeding. I was heartbroken but that was clearly his time. I had no idea how to stop breastfeeding and I didn't want to, but children let you know when they're ready and it's important to respect that.

Breastfeeding Henry was one of the toughest, easiest and most rewarding things I have ever done. I think it also pulled me out of my depression in hindsight (that's how powerful it was for me). Being a midwife definitely did not give me an advantage over everyone else. On the contrary, I know many a midwife who stopped breastfeeding because of lack of support, it was too painful, or they just didn't like it. If anyone ever tells you that they found breastfeeding easy then rest assured, they are a minority. Most women experience various struggles with breastfeeding. What I learned from my journey is that the early days are brutal! As well as the physical problems I encountered, I never anticipated the mental ones (breastfeeding is 90 per cent mental). No training ever covered that for me. I didn't have the reassurance of seeing Henry drink a set amount of milk from a bottle, I just had to trust that he was getting that from my breasts. While relentlessly checking for wet and dirty nappies for reassurance, counting down the days until I could get him weighed again and panicking that every time he cried, it could have been because he was hungry because maybe my boobs weren't giving him enough.

If you want to breastfeed, you can't do it alone. You need a community of equally supportive people around you who won't tell you at every hurdle to give the baby a bottle. You need to call upon your midwives, health visitors, community services (health visitors know who to contact in your area), social media groups, friends or family who have breastfed. It can be very lonely breast-feeding in the early days so ask for help. Please don't suffer in silence. I look back at my journey now and I think breastfeeding is a little bit like learning to drive. The first six weeks are where you have to do everything by the rules, such as position and attachment, to ensure you get established in your feeding. After six weeks is when you pass your test and that's when you really learn to breastfeed. You and baby get confident with each other. You know how your bodies work, which positions you prefer, which boob baby prefers, and you trust that you can do this.

Sian Munt

If anyone had asked me ten years ago if I would breast-feed, I would have replied no way! No way would I be confident enough to feed my baby in front of others, the thought of someone looking at me would send my anxiety through the roof. Everything changed when I came under the influence of Chantelle, my cousin, sharing her breastfeeding journey on Instagram. I just remember how it saddened me to see how she was met with so much negativity with her decision to breastfeed her twins but how amazing that she proved everyone who doubted her wrong. Why SHOULD we care about what others think? No one has the right to judge any-one! I felt empowered, I WANTED to breastfeed my baby so I would.

Our own journey began when Ada was born via emergency caesarean section after two long days and two long nights of labour. I was devastated that I couldn't have the natural water birth that I'd dreamt of, I really felt like I had let myself down even though there was nothing different or more I could have done. I think I put far too much pressure on myself to have a 'natural' birth. My thoughts then were if I can't birth my baby naturally, I was sure as anything going to feed her naturally, my body would not let me down again. I have never felt more determined and passionate about something before, I didn't even think that I could have such focus! Ada had to have an IV drip put in almost immediately after birth and a dose of antibiotics as I had developed a temperature during labour. Once done, we got to have our 'Golden Hour'. Ada latched on with support from my midwife and began feeding. I was wheeled to a private room and the midwives there checked her latch and said that she knew exactly what she was doing. I felt so proud. We spent the next two days in hospital and feeding continued to go well.

We'd been home a couple of days when I woke up during the night after being asleep for an hour or so feeling feverish. I remember being quite disorientated and shivering uncontrollably and I struggled to get up from the bed. I had to get Danny (my partner) to pull me up and help me to the toilet, I went back to sleep and felt fine when I got up for Ada's next feed. The same thing happened the following night. The midwife came over the next morning and I mentioned it, she explained that it was my milk coming in and it can give you flu-like symptoms.

The following day, I lay on the sofa and I just didn't feel right. I checked my temperature and it was high so I took some paracetamol. After half an hour, I checked it again and it had risen. My gut was telling me to call the midwife. She came over to the house to check me over. Shortly after arriving, she called the hospital and advised I go in and asked me to pack a bag just in case. Ada, Danny and I got to the hospital and I had some blood tests, which confirmed I had sepsis. I was immediately put on an IV drip of antibiotics. Within a couple of minutes, I felt extremely sick and dizzy, then my skin was unbelievably itchy. Danny called for help and all I remember was the room filled with people. I was laid on the bed and had an oxygen mask over my face. I'd had an anaphylactic shock (a severe allergic reaction) to the antibiotics. All I could think about was that Ada needed a feed very soon! Once antihistamine was put through my IV and the reaction began to calm, I pulled the mask down and said, 'Can I still feed my baby?' The nurse smiled and said, 'Don't worry about that now, we'll work something out!'

The nurses helped me express so Danny would be able to feed her during the night. I remember having a pump on each boob and within a few minutes, both bottles were filled to the top! The nurses were amazed by my supply and said we could make pancakes with it! When I got to ICU, the nurses there were fantastic and said they didn't have a problem with Danny bringing Ada to me so I could continue to feed. I continued to pump throughout the night to keep up my supply.

We continued to breastfeed exclusively and five months later, we are still going strong. I am loving every moment and the bond I feel between my daughter and I is indescribable. Breastfeeding really is my biggest ever achievement and I feel so proud to be able to nurture my baby myself, it really does give you this overwhelming feeling of power!

Charlotte Galbally

As a new mother of five, I was adamant and passionate about breastfeeding my final child. Henry, my firstborn, who is now six and a half, was exclusively breastfed from when he was about ten minutes old until he was about a year old. I enjoyed every moment and loved that it created a wonderful mother and baby bond.

Baby number two would have followed suit However, baby number two turned into baby number two, three and four, as we had beautiful triplet girls. It took me a while to persuade myself during the pregnancy that it would be OK not to breastfeed them, but once they were born, I started off adamant that I would and for the first eight weeks I tried with every ounce of strength

I had. Unfortunately, I had a complication and a reaction to the clexane injection (post C-section medication to thin blood after the operation) and my milk was unusable for the first week, once it came in on day 5. I managed to hand express for the first five days to give the girls the colostrum, but then until day 12, I had to 'pump and dump', which was soul-destroying, to be brutally honest. Due to the fact my milk wasn't usable, the girls were on feeding tubes and were given SMA® Gold preterm milk. This at the time hurt me emotionally and mentally as I felt I was letting the babies down when they needed my milk the most.

Once the medication was out of my system, I managed to express my milk and give it to the girls through bottle or tube, but due to the milk being split into three, it was topped up with the formula to ensure the girls were hitting their milk target per day to gain weight and hopefully get them out of neonatal and home.

At around eight weeks, I found looking after three newborn babies plus Henry (who was four) after my husband Alex had gone back to work a struggle. Through the advice of my family and medical professionals and against my will slightly, I gave up breastfeeding the girls. I never thought I would give up and it made me feel like a failure. It took me some time to come to terms with it, but looking back, it was the right decision for me. I knew exactly how much milk they were getting, it took the pressure off me and allowed Alex to be more hands-on, and it made me feel less exhausted and gave me more time to be the mum my children needed. I'm still proud of myself and I know in my heart I gave it as much as I could.

As I write this, Jimmy has joined the family and he is five months old. I have pretty much replicated what I did with Henry. I have really found myself loving breastfeeding – I have exclusively breastfed apart from a few bottles, which family has carried out when I've expressed my milk, and the family has managed to be involved and feed him by bottle.

My biggest challenge was breastfeeding a newborn, Jimmy, with four other children! The first few days I was in hospital it was bliss. Once I got home the challenges began. Henry understood and gave me some time and space when it was feeding time, but the girls were difficult – when Jimmy was born, they were two and a half years old, at the peak of being toddlers! When I would sit and need to feed him, they all wanted to be part of it, which sounds very sweet but it was a nightmare! They would all want to sit with me, on my head pretty much. I felt this was so difficult for little Jimmy to have the calm and quiet to learn how to feed – it was new to him, new to me again, and he needed to be able to have that time to learn to latch on and feed properly without constant distractions. But I had to learn to manage this; I didn't want to push them away and make them feel like they were not part of it, I didn't want to create a problem or a divide by saying they can't be close when I am feeding.

The first few days at home was really tough. Alex was brilliant and would be very hands-on with the children so I could dedicate my time to Jimmy and giving him my boob as and when he wanted milk. I felt totally overwhelmed by everything and everyone. All I wanted was to sit on the sofa and feed my new baby boy. The girls had started to bicker and push and shove about who could sit the closest to me and baby. But it just wasn't working and I felt harassed and stressed, and this was rubbing off on Jimmy. It was at that point that I thought, *What am I doing, how am I going to make breastfeeding work, should I give up and bottle feed?* I knew something had to change, but I wanted it to be a positive effect for the family, I didn't want to have to take myself off on my own to feed.

So, we made 'feeding time' a big deal. Alex would take the children out to the garden or to the playroom to play while I was feeding. Feeding time also meant calm and a quiet time for everyone else, so we would all sit down together and watch something on TV. As time went on, Jimmy settled into more of a routine so I would try my hardest to work this around meals, so all the children would be sitting down at the table eating and occupied, and I could sit near them, feeding. I would say if you are in the middle of trying to breastfeed a newborn and you have other children and think this is impossible, it's not! You just have to figure out what works best for you and your family, how you can distract the older children while feeding, making sure an older child feels included and not pushed away. It can be done and a lot of it is pure determination and dedication.

Evelynda Collison

When I found out I was pregnant, there was never a doubt in my mind that I was going to breastfeed my baby – even when I found out I was having twins, I never questioned how I would feed them. I naively thought it wouldn't be much more difficult than one and regardless there wasn't any alternative in my mind for me. In my opinion, from what I know about breastfeeding, it is what is best for me and my babies.

My mum was a midwife and is now a senior lecturer in midwifery for a university, so I had the best teacher and source of support when I had questions. I didn't listen to people who thought that they were being supportive by telling me it's OK to quit and give them a bottle before I'd even started; of course it's OK to quit, but I was determined to make it work and what I needed was support. I vaguely remember the first time I breastfed Hayden and Hendrix, although I wouldn't really call it breastfeeding – I was completely 'out of it' after pushing for hours and just remember seeing the midwife holding my boob to my tiny baby's mouth, as I couldn't physically do it myself. Once I was able to hold them and try to feed them myself, it was nothing like I'd been taught. I had no idea what I was doing and it was hard getting them to latch on. Suddenly, you're all alone in the postnatal ward with your babies and you've gone from having so much attention from so many midwives to basically figuring it out alone. I didn't know when I should be feeding them and I definitely hadn't mastered how – I really thought it would be something that would come naturally to me. It didn't, and I don't think it does for anyone.

One of my main worries was milk production, but my amazing midwife recommended I hand-express colostrum 14 days before my induction to help lessen any stress I may feel in hospital if I was unable to feed the twins. This tip was invaluable as we were in hospital for a few days and sometimes the boys wouldn't feed. We couldn't really go home until they did, so I'd feed them my colostrum out of a syringe just to ensure they were getting enough. Another fear I had was the babies becoming underweight and having to go back to hospital in the first couple of weeks. As amazing as the staff and midwives were, I did not want to go back into hospital ever again – we had spent five days there.

The boys were also jaundiced and breastfeeding is a great way to flush it out of their system, so that was another motivator. Luckily my milk came in on the third day and I think that was mainly due to the colostrum collection I'd done before their arrival. Other than those initial concerns, I never worried that my babies weren't getting enough milk. I heard time and time again the unfounded belief that a breastfed baby isn't getting enough milk because you can't see how much they're taking in: 'If you haven't made up a bottle to a certain amount of ounces how do you know how much they're getting?' I didn't know, but I knew that my babies knew when they were full and that's when they stopped feeding. I never felt the urge to top up with formula because I felt that the baby instinctively eats as much as they want, not as much as you want them to eat. Don't get me wrong – I still had a little panic every time the health visitor came to weigh them, in fear of the possibility that they may have lost weight (they will do in their first week).

I use my breast milk for more than just feeding my babies – the stuff is like liquid gold. My babies have quite bad eczema and I've used my milk for milk baths, which does wonders for their skin. They come out the bath so silky smooth and barely scratching. I've also mixed it in with moisturisers for the same reason. I use it for lots of things. I absolutely love breastfeeding. The bond it's formed between me and my babies is indescribable. It makes me feel so proud because breastfeeding is so hard – SO, SO HARD – and I'm very lucky that I was able to make a success of it and that I had the support from my friends and family to do so. I do wish someone had told me how hard it was going to be, how taxing it is on your mind and your body, how time consuming it is and how it takes over the whole of your life so much that you can't really do anything but breastfeed. It was definitely the best choice I could have made and I only have positive things to say about it.

Breastfeeding Dates for the Diary

Black Breastfeeding Awareness Week

Black Breastfeeding Awareness Week is on August 25th to 31st every year and is an important week. It was originally founded in the US to raise awareness about the racial disparity in breastfeeding rates[1]. Black women have a complex cultural history around breastfeeding. Slavery in the US was only officially abolished in December 1885, which is less than 200 hundred years ago. Before this time, black women and mothers were often forced to become wet nurses to nourish and care for their white enslaver's babies[2]. There is a lot of trauma surrounding breastfeeding stemming from this history, which I learnt has been passed down in the black community.

In the UK, black women are five times more likely to die in childbirth than white women, and black infants also have a higher mortality rate than any other ethnicity.

The benefits of breastfeeding are not only for babies but for mums too[3]. Breastfeeding can help protect children from diseases that are more common in black communities, including upper respiratory infections, type 2 diabetes, asthma and childhood obesity, all of which breastfeeding is known to protect against[4].

There is also a huge lack of diversity in the lactation field, and so this week is a time to highlight and celebrate the breastfeeding champions in the black community.

---

[1] http://blackbreastfeedingweek.org/why-we-need-black-breastfeeding-week/

[2] https://www.upworthy.com/its-black-breastfeeding-week-if-you-wonder-why-this-gut-punching-poem-offers-one-reason

[3] https://www.breastfeedingnetwork.org.uk/guest-blog-by-ruth-dennison-why-black-breastfeeding-week

[4] https://www.scarymommy.com/black-breastfeeding-week-is-crucial/

This is Sylvia Udomhiaye's story:

'I breastfed my first child until he was 19 months old and my second until she was 17 months. This was mainly for two reasons: one, because I enjoyed the bonding time it gave us and two, probably out of rebellion to the unwritten rules of breastfeeding in the African culture. I say African because I'm Nigerian, so can only speak for that side.

When I had my first child, I was all set to breastfeed exclusively and was very excited. I got home on day one and the families came over to visit. The first thing I was told is that I'd have to formula feed because if I only gave my son breastmilk he wouldn't be full, and that at least with formula I could get a good night's sleep. I was adamant that I wasn't going to give him formula, but then I started to feel the pressure. I started to feel like a bad mum, thinking I wasn't giving my child enough food and was, in effect, starving him. Every time he cried after a feed I was met with disapproving looks and comments – they acted like I wasn't allowing him to get enough food due to my own selfish needs. I tried to shrug those feelings off.

The following day there were at least three visitors telling me I'd need to give my baby formula or he'd be hungry. I sat in a chair in tears, feeling helpless, and I gave in. My son hiccupped and I was also told off for not giving him water, it was silly not to give him water they said, so they pretty much demanded and I gave in to that too.

Over time, I noticed that I started giving him formula less and less because I felt like a right had been taken away from me. I was trying to regain some form of control. By the time my baby was six months old he was pretty much exclusively breastfed again. I regained some form of control back but then the older he got the disapproving looks returned:

"Surely he's too old to be breastfed?" "When are you going to stop?".

Once he hit 12 months I really got it, it was like I was supposed to stop overnight ("He's far too old now!"), but I persevered. I wasn't going to let myself feel how I did in the beginning. I felt like I was doing what was best for my baby. One day my boob was leaking and one of my Auntie's noticed, and she said, "Are you still breastfeeding?" She was so shocked that he was still being breastfed after one. I felt so embarrassed. I persevered through this and carried on until he was 19 months. I'm really happy I did, but I shouldn't have had to go through everything I did just because I decided to exclusively breastfeed my baby. It made the whole experience so tense and almost traumatic for me, when I should have been enjoying such a special moment. I was able to persevere because despite all this I have relatively thick skin and can be a bit stubborn. For someone else, this may not be the case, so people need to educate themselves on the benefits of breastfeeding before putting someone off as this could be detrimental to mum and baby.

I've just had my third baby and, although it's been a horrible time in 2020 with everything that's going on in the world, having my baby during the pandemic lockdown has been the best thing for me. No prying eyes, no pressure, just me and my baby. And I tell you, breastfeeding has felt amazing. I've even enjoyed waking up at all hours of the night just to breastfeed. One thing that needs to change is the perception that breastfeeding isn't enough – it is enough, and things have changed since 20-plus years ago.'

World Breastfeeding Week

World Breastfeeding Week is celebrated every year from 1st to 7th August, to encourage breastfeeding and improve the health of babies around the world. Its purpose is to highlight the importance of breastfeeding and all of the health benefits for baby and mother, to help empower and encourage women. There is a different theme each year to shine a spotlight on different areas of breastfeeding.

National Breastfeeding Week

This falls in June and is a different week each year, and it also celebrates different themes each time. This is a great time to provide an opportunity to look at the support women currently receive and what might be improved, and to reflect on the many benefits of breastfeeding and why it is something so worth celebrating.

Breastfeeding Awareness Month

The month of August is breastfeeding awareness month. Here are some ways to observe and take part.

- Learn: learn new things about breastfeeding you might not have known before. Research and read articles.
- Advocate: be an advocate for a breastfeeding mum. Breastfeeding mums can come up against criticism in work, in public, from friends and family, so become their cheerleader and support network.
- Share: share your own experiences and knowledge, online or with friends, to help normalise and put an end to any stigmas around breastfeeding.

Support

Helplines

I appreciate this isn't face-to-face support – which is best, I find – but you can get advice and support from people that you know are fully qualified and going to give you the correct information, with the main goal of helping you breastfeed your baby:

Association of Breastfeeding Mothers (ABM)
0300 330 5453
www.abm.me.uk

La Leche League
0345 120 2918
www.laleche.org.uk

National Breastfeeding Helpline
0300 100 0212
www.nationalbreastfeedinghelpline.org.uk

National Childbirth Trust (NCT)
0300 330 0700
www.nct.org.uk

Face-to-face support

Midwives and health visitors can give you help and advice. They may be able to help you with any problems or questions you have, but if you are not happy with the information that has been presented to you, then please request some face-to-face support from a lactation consultant, breastfeeding specialist or infant feeding coordinator. Remember to always go with your gut.

Find a local breastfeeding support group. Ask your midwife or health visitor for any groups they know of. You can also contact the National Breastfeeding Helpline (see page 249), who can let you know of any local groups.

In the UK there are different levels of support:

1. Peer supporters: They have their own personal experiences of breastfeeding and some training from one of the voluntary organisations (listed overleaf), they will pass more complex problems on to a breastfeeding counsellor or IBCLC.
2. Breastfeeding councillors: They are trained and accredited by the four voluntary organisations (Association of Breastfeeding Mothers, Breastfeeding Network, La Leche League or NCT). They have breastfed their own babies and have undertaken comprehensive part-time training for two to three years.
3. IBCLC Lactation Consultant: The professional level of qualification in breastfeeding assistance. They undergo extensive training, and have to put in 1000 hours of clinical practice in the five years prior to being able to apply for the exam.

Internet support

I cannot recommend this enough if I tried! The Breastfeeding Twins and Triplets Facebook group was the best support on my breastfeeding journey. The advice and knowledge from professionals and experienced mums was second to none and getting help after a few taps of a finger was invaluable to me – if you are busy, can't plan a phone call or physically drop in to a group, this is so handy and efficient. I have not been a part of the Facebook group for singleton babies, but it comes highly recommended and is called UK Breastfeeding Support. There are also the UK Relactation and Adoptive Breastfeeding Support and Breastfeeding Older Babies and Beyond Facebook groups. Please read all Facebook group's guidelines carefully before joining.

As soon as you find out you are pregnant, add yourselves to these Facebook groups, start stocking up on knowledge and then, once your baby arrives, they will be there for you with support and advice if any problems arise.

The Breastfeeding Network
www.breastfeedingnetwork.org.uk

Lactation Consultants of Great Britain
www.lcgb.org

UNICEF UK Baby Friendly Initiative
www.unicef.org.uk/babyfriendly

Association of Tongue-Tie Practitioners
www.tongue-tie.org.uk

Adoption UK
www.adoptionuk.org

Fertility Network UK
www.fertilitynetworkuk.org

LGBT Foundation
www.lgbt.foundation/

Acknowledgements

First of all, I would like to give a big thank you to each and every woman that has ever contacted me, asking me for help and advice on breastfeeding. Had it not been for you, I may not have known about the passion, drive and desire I had inside me to help women to breastfeed. You and all of my online followers gave me the courage and confidence to share my breastfeeding journey online, and to write this book on breastfeeding in the first place. I will forever be eternally grateful.

I would like to thank my editor Beth at Blink. From the moment I met her, I knew she was my woman! She has such a passion for wanting to help women write books to help support other women and I couldn't think of a better person to work alongside me. We both have the same vision of the ultimate end goal, with that one person in mind: the reader, the new mum. I am so incredibly lucky to have had her by my side writing this book.

My birthing midwife Amanda, who helped me latch Twin 2, Blakely, when I was still being stitched up from my C-section. I found my birth with the twins very traumatic, but Amanda was my shining light through the darkness of the tough times. I remember she did not let go of my hand. She stayed with me even when her shift had finished to make sure me and the girls were OK, something I will never forget or be grateful enough for.

The MSW Maternity support worker on the ward, Suzanne, thoroughly looked after me, the girls and my husband Lewis.

The care she gave us will stay with me forever – we had a few hospital admissions on the children's ward and another on the postnatal ward, and every time Suzanne would come and visit, and help with my breastfeeding journey after seeing how important it was for me.

My grandad was one of my biggest supporters in life and, heartbreakingly, he passed away when the twins were just four weeks old. But he has still been my constant guiding light throughout writing this book. I had a lot of self-doubt and moments when I thought, *I cannot do this*, and he would always pop into my mind and I would wonder what he would say to me. I shook off any negative thoughts and knew I could do this.

My wonderful husband Lewis, mum Zelda and sister Nikita, who have given me nothing but amazing support throughout my breastfeeding journeys and in writing this book. If it was not for the support of these three, would I have breastfed for as long? Maybe not, but all I know is having the full support from them all gave me the confidence to feed my children the way I wanted, and for how long I wanted to.

Another thank you goes to the family members who mocked me for breastfeeding for so long and for suggesting why I wanted to breastfeed my twins. You gave me the drive to prove you wrong and also showed me how many narrow-minded people there are still in the world when it comes to breastfeeding. You have helped my mission to educate and give the passion and drive to as many women as possible to feed their babies how they want to, not how other people think they should.

* * *

I want to end this book with one final thank you to you – thank you for reading this book. I have really gone through every emotion you can think of writing it. I have cried, writing my story and thinking about how my mental health was affected. My blood has boiled, writing about interfering family members, not only for myself but for all the women who will also have that same fight on their hands. I have laughed while reading back some things I put in here (which I hadn't even remembered writing!). I have felt completely proud, throughout my whole body, reading the stories of other mums (and one dad) on their breastfeeding journeys. And I have felt the passion flow through my veins for hopefully being able to help you with your breastfeeding journey.

I want you to remember that if you decide that actually breastfeeding is not for you, that's OK, you do YOU! If you do decide to give breastfeeding a go and then change your mind, that's also OK. And if you are struggling, do not feel ashamed to contact someone for support. Make sure you are kind to yourself and always trust your gut!

Thank you so much once again. You will never understand the gratitude I have for every person who has taken the time to read my words. I'm crying again, so this is goodbye for now!

Chantelle x

Resources & Bibliography

Books

Evans, Kate, *The Food of Love: Your Formula for Successful Breastfeeding*, Myriad 2008

La Leche League International, *The Womanly Art of Breastfeeding*, Pinter & Martin 2010

Mathur, Anna, *Mind Over Mother: Every mum's guide to worry and anxiety in the first year*, Piatkus 2020

Pickett, Emma, *You've Got it in You: A Positive Guide to Breast Feeding*, Matador 2016

Websites

www.kellymom.com
www.NCT.org.uk
www.NHS.uk
www.breastfedbabies.org
www.emmasdiary.co.uk
www.nct.org.uk
www.babycentre.co.uk
www.laleche.org.uk
www.breastfeedingnetwork.org.uk

Index